I would like to dedicate this book to my three beautiful new grandchildren, Ella, Alessia and Lily. They are three very special angels.
I am very proud to be their grandfather.

The Author

John McKenna is a scientist and a retired medical doctor who has been practising natural medicine for 25 years. He is the bestselling author of *Antibiotics, Good Food, Hard to Stomach, Natural Alternatives to Antibiotics* and *Alternatives to Tranquillisers*. He lives in Wexford.

What You Can Do to Prevent Cancer

John McKenna BA, MB ChB

Gill & Macmillan

Gill & Macmillan
Hume Avenue, Park West, Dublin 12
www.gillmacmillanbooks.ie

© John McKenna 2015
978 07171 6110 2

Typography design by Make Communication
Print origination by Carole Lynch
Index compiled by Eileen O'Neill
Printed and bound by ScandBook AB, Sweden

This book is typeset in Linotype Minion and Neue Helvetica.

The paper used in this book comes from the wood pulp of
managed forests. For every tree felled, at least one tree is
planted, thereby renewing natural resources.

A CIP catalogue record for this book is available
from the British Library.

5 4 3 2 1

The author and publisher have made every effort to trace
all copyright holders, but if any has been inadvertently
overlooked we would be pleased to make the necessary
arrangements at the first opportunity.

Contents

Acknowledgements

I would like to thank Fergal Tobin and Nicki Howard for agreeing to publish this book, and all the editorial staff at Gill & Macmillan, especially my commissioning editor, Deirdre Nolan, for their help in turning the manuscript into this wonderful book. I would also like to acknowledge the great support and help provided by my publishers over the past twenty-five years. I wish you many blessings.

A big thanks to all my patients in Ireland and abroad. I am indebted to all of you as I have learned so much from you all.

A massive thanks to my parents, who helped to shape me into the person I am today. I think about both of you all the time and I am sad that we did not have more time together while you were still alive.

I am especially grateful to my four children, Charity, Jackie, Marianne and David. You have been very supportive and helpful. I am very proud of all of you.

I am particularly grateful to my son, David, for setting up a Facebook page for me (www.facebook.com/nutritionmed) and for constructing a website (still being built) to allow me access to a much wider audience. Well done!

Introduction

After heart disease, cancer has become the second leading cause of death in the Western world. However, many people have lived on this planet and not succumbed to cancer. There are still population groups around the world in which the cancer rate is very low or zero. Admittedly, most of these groups have little contact with Western civilisation.

However, even if you live smack bang in the middle of a Western city, you can still minimise your risk of developing cancer. In other words, it is entirely possible to prevent cancer from taking hold in your body. All that is required is for you to become aware of the root causes of cancer and how to reduce your risk. Creating such awareness is the purpose of this book.

I have written this book with the purpose of showing you that most cancers are completely preventable. From this I exclude cancers due to genetic factors. But since only five to ten per cent of cancers are genetic, it follows that 90 to 95 per cent can be avoided. Drawing on scientific and medical research, this book will describe what adjustments you need to make to your lifestyle in order to protect yourself.

It is not exposure to individual carcinogens, or substances that can cause cancer, such as pesticides in food that dictates whether you will develop cancer. Rather, it's the ability of your immune system to protect you that decides your fate.

A factor that has a pronounced weakening effect on your immunity is stress. Most people who develop cancer have had ongoing stress in their lives prior to the diagnosis.

If you combine ongoing or previous stress with exposure to carcinogens and a Western diet rich in processed foods, the likelihood of developing cancer increases significantly. The main aim of this book is to highlight simple things that you can do to boost your defence against cancer.

First, in Chapter 1, we will look at why cancer is essentially a Western disease. Chapter 2 deals with the less well-known carcinogens in your immediate environment, while Chapter 3 examines the dangerous substances in the food and drink you put into your body every day. Chapter 4 highlights the role of the gut in a healthy immune system and how gut problems can be rectified. Chapters 5 and 6 examine diet and food in specific detail, including foods to avoid and foods with anti-cancer properties, while Chapter 7 gives advice on where to buy your food. I look at the critical issue of stress in Chapter 8 and provide practical advice on overcoming stress, including simple exercises you can do. Chapter 9 is an overview of the role of obesity in cancer. The book concludes with a chapter containing practical advice for the avoidance/treatment of specific cancers.

If you follow the advice in this book, you stand an excellent chance of avoiding cancer. If you pass it on to your children and relatives you will be helping your family and community at large. Following this advice means you can start preventing cancer right away. There is no need to wait for some magic pill because the power lies with you. You can take control by eliminating harmful elements in your environment, altering your diet, boosting your immunity and overcoming your stress.

Recently I read that a number of cancers are the result of bad luck and have nothing to do with diet, poor gut health or stress. If this truly were the case, then the rates of these cancers would have been as high historically, and people such as the Inuit of Greenland and the Sami of northern Scandinavia would have similar incidences.

There is as much misinformation out there as there is information. There are vested interests at work whose aim it is to confuse you. I'm referring in particular to drug companies, food manufacturers and politicians. Be skeptical about everything you hear, *see* or read about cancer, including material based on scientific and medical research, especially industry-funded research. Before reading any article I always check first to *see* who funded the research. If it is a drug company or other industry I tend to discard it.

However, even government-funded research, which makes use of public funds, can be biased. Two eminent professors, one from Harvard Medical School and the other from Stanford Medical School in the us, have been accused of carrying out illegal drug trials while using public funds to conduct their research. Both of these professors had strong financial links to the drug companies that manufactured the drugs used in these illicit trials (Campbell *et al.* 2007).

I would urge you to take charge of your own life and not be dependent on the system to help you. If you implement even some of the measures I have outlined, you should notice an improvement in your overall health. Always keep in mind the fact that Nature is there to assist you.

I wish you and your loved ones excellent health so that you get full enjoyment out of living.

JOHN McKENNA
March 2015

Chapter 1
Cancer is a Western Disease

Many parts of the developing world have major health problems but cancer is not one of them. I worked on and off between 1977 and 2002 in different parts of Africa and, during my time there, I observed three population groups with three different disease spectrums – the rural Africans, the white settlers and the urban Africans.

The rural African very occasionally presented with cancer but this was cancer associated with chronic infections. In southern Africa (Zimbabwe, Botswana, Namibia, Lesotho and South Africa), for example, hepatitis B can progress to cause chronic active hepatitis, which is an infection of the liver that can ultimately result in primary liver cancer. In medical school, we were taught that primary liver cancer occurred in only two parts of the world – southern Africa and South-East Asia – where the carrier rate for hepatitis B is very high. Common cancers such as breast, prostate and colon cancer were rare or absent in rural Africans.

Over the years, the British, French, Germans, Portuguese, Belgians, Dutch and others colonised various parts of Africa. Many of these white European settlers lived a Western lifestyle and ate a Western diet. In this population group the disease pattern was very different: cancer was remarkably common.

However, once Africans moved to the cities and began to eat a Western diet, refined carbohydrates in particular, and suffer the stresses of a modern lifestyle, they became more susceptible to cancer. They represented a transitional population group who still presented with a disease spectrum similar to their rural relatives, but the longer they spent in urban areas the more their disease pattern resembled that of the white folk.

Back in the 1970s and 1980s, when the incidence of cancer increased quite markedly, especially in the USA, UK and Continental Europe, cancer was described by many as the disease of the affluent. The only type of cancer found in less developed areas of the world was that associated with a chronic infection, such as primary liver cancer. This type of cancer was referred to as the poor man's cancer.

THE RISE IN CANCER

Since 1940 the incidence of cancer has increased in all major industrialised countries. Figure 1.1 shows the marked rise in breast cancer as an example.

As you can *see*, in 1940 the incidence of breast cancer in the USA was approximately 40 per 100,000 of the population or, put another way, 4 in every 10,000 people developed the disease. By 1970, this had doubled to 80 per 100,000; by 2000, it had risen to 120 per 100,000.

When you compare these figures with those of China, for example, the difference is very marked. However, once the Chinese migrate to Western countries, their chance of developing cancer increases (Servan-Schreiber, 2011).

Figure 1.1: *Breast Cancer Incidence in USA, 1940–2000*

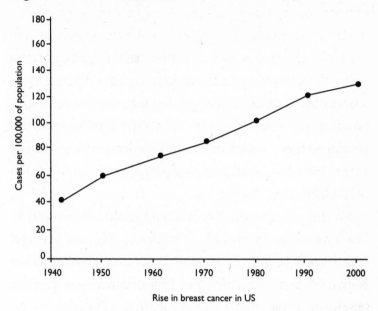

Rise in breast cancer in US

Source: Quoted in McGrath, K.G., 'An earlier age of breast cancer diagnosis related to more frequent use of antiperspirants/ deodorants and underarm shaving', *European Journal of Cancer Prevention*, 12(6), 2003: 480.

The incidence of prostate cancer has risen even faster still.

Many experts in the field are calling this an epidemic of cancer in the West.

When I was at medical school many moons ago we were taught that cancer for the most part affected the very young and the elderly because the immune system was not well developed in the young and was less efficient in the elderly. Since the mid-1970s, this pattern has changed very dramatically. Now any age group can be affected. It is not uncommon for fifty-year-olds and even forty-year-olds to test positive for cancer. I was shocked the first time I saw breast cancer in a woman aged thirty-five. She was under the care of an oncologist, but after having had a mastectomy she refused to take chemotherapy and opted to come to *see* me.

Also, the type of cancer *see*n in younger age groups tends to be faster growing and more virulent. For example, prostate cancer in an eighty-year-old tends to be quite slow growing and often the man will die of other causes, but prostate cancer in a fifty-year-old tends to be much more aggressive and is more likely to kill.

It is clear that the dynamics of this disease have altered significantly. Not only is it increasing in incidence and so affecting many more people, it is also creeping into younger and younger age groups and presenting a much more aggressive picture. There must be an explanation for this phenomenon.

A major research study, published in the journal *Science* in 2003, showed that the risk of getting breast cancer before the age of fifty has tripled for women born after the Second World War compared to the risk for women born before the war (King, 2003). Other studies show a similar pattern for other cancers. These studies suggest that the problem began around the time of the Second World War. So something quite significant changed in the 1940s/early 1950s.

In 2000 a research article published in the *New England Journal of Medicine* stated that many lines of evidence indicate that the factors that determine the great majority of cancers are largely exogenous (external) and thus preventable. These include factors related to lifestyle as well as toxins in food, air and water (Lichenstein *et al.*, 2000). If we alter our lifestyle, especially our diet, and clean up our immediate environment, we stand a good chance of fending off up to 80 per cent of cancers. This is an incredible admission that the war on cancer should be fought on the basis of educating people about altering their lifestyle and about the sources of toxicity in the environment to avoid.

More money should be spent on preventive medicine. The truth is that there is no profit to be made in preventive medicine and so it would not attract private funding. Since Western scientific and medical research is dependent on funding from the drug companies, most research is directed towards finding some miracle cancer drug that can be patented to serve the insatiable appetite for profit. Politicians are also dependent on drug companies for taxes and for the employment of their citizens, so there is little political will to fund preventive medicine.

Therefore, once again it is up to you, the reader, to take responsibility for your own health and to educate yourself in how to prevent cancer. If you do this you have an excellent chance of avoiding cancer. You will also have much better health and get more out of life.

Before we look at what changed in the 1940s to bring about such an increase in the incidence of cancer, I would like to outline how cancer develops within the body, and to illustrate the role of lifestyle and environmental factors in this process.

THE ORIGINS AND DEVELOPMENT OF CANCER
Cancer Comes from Within

Some people believe that cancer is something that comes from outside your body and attacks you. They believe that cancer is like influenza or MRSA in that you contract it and it takes hold in your body and harms you – like some gruesome monster in a horror movie.

The truth is rather different. The creation of cancer cells is a normal natural process that occurs every day in your body. It is what happens when things go awry in the natural process of cell division, a process by which a parent cell divides into two or more daughter cells. Cells in your body multiply every day in an effort to replace old cells or to repair a wound, for example. As with any process, things can go wrong. When this happens, an abnormal cell is produced which we call a cancer cell.

In most cases this is not a problem as your immune system will detect it and dispose of it rapidly. Our immune cells, especially a particular type of white blood cell called natural killer cells (a very appropriate name), take care of these abnormal cells by destroying them. They are the special forces of the immune system. Therefore, every day your body produces cancer cells and every day your immune system deals with them. Now you can *see* how foolish it is to think of cancer as some alien from outer space or some monster from the dark side of the moon coming to attack you. So the real reason why cancer can occur and be allowed to take hold in your body is because your immune system has been weakened. It is more accurate to view cancer as a malfunction of the immune system. This is why cancer used to occur only in the elderly and the very young because, as I explained earlier, the immune system is not well developed in the very young and is going downhill in the elderly.

There is a wonderful example of the role of the immune system in protecting the body against cancer from tests done on laboratory mice. To study cancer, scientists inject high doses of cancer cells into the bodies of lab mice. The high doses of cancer cells are to ensure that the animals consequently develop the disease and therefore can be used for cancer research. (Thousands of mice, rats, guinea pigs and other animals suffer and die at the hands of medical science every day around the world.)

In 2002 something very strange happened in a lab at Wake Forest University, North Carolina: one of the mice that had been injected with the standard dose of cancer cells did not develop cancer. This was a great surprise to the researcher. She consulted with her supervisor, who suggested using double the dosage. Still the mouse showed no signs of developing cancer. The researcher then injected ten times the dosage, sure that this would do the trick. Still the mouse did not develop cancer. They had found a mouse that was most unusual in that it was resistant to cancer. They named him 'Mighty Mouse' (Cui, 2003).

Mighty Mouse had a very strong immune system that enabled him to mount a powerful immune response once the cancer cells were injected into his body. This is a very important message to keep at the forefront of your mind when reading the rest of this book.

Preventing cancer is fundamentally all about finding ways to avoid harming the immune system and to strengthen immunity. In particular, if you strengthen your immune system and avoid too much exposure to harmful agents in your environment, you will be able to take care of whatever cancer cells arise in your body on an ongoing basis. You can become like Mighty Mouse.

From now on, view cancer as a natural process that happens every day in every one of us and that will not develop into anything sinister if our immunity is in top form.

How Are Cancer Cells Different?

Cancer cells are abnormal cells and behave abnormally. They do not obey the rules that normal cells follow. Cancer cells can be thought of as rogue cells running amok and creating havoc in the body.

An amazing control system operates in your body. This control system operates at all levels, from the control of essential nutrient levels to the control of individual cells. For example, if the water level in your bloodstream decreases, the thirst centre in your brain is triggered to tell you to drink more water. Similarly, when you cut your skin with a knife, skin cells are triggered to multiply to replace those that have been damaged. But this multiplication, also called cell division, stops when a sufficient number of cells have been made. So, there are triggers that initiate cell division and triggers that stop it, in the same way that your sensation of thirst is initiated and then stopped, once you drink enough water.

With cancer cells, the same control system does not function correctly and so cancer cells multiply in an out-of-control manner, creating abnormal lumps and bumps. This is sometimes referred to as cell division gone mad.

Normal cells that are damaged beyond repair by cuts, bruises and so on are triggered by the body's control system to die. This is a normal, natural process that allows the body to remove cells that are no longer of any use. With cancer cells, this normal process does not work. So damaged cells are not removed and may harm neighbouring normal cells.

Normal cells derive their energy mainly from glucose. This glucose is broken down into energy in the mitochondria of the cell, a process that is dependent on oxygen. Glucose is also the main source of energy in cancer cells, but it is not only broken down in the mitochondria but also in the main body of the cell, and the process is not dependent on oxygen. Cancer cells consume very large amounts of glucose compared to normal cells. This is a very important point to remember when you wish to prevent or treat cancer. If cancer is deprived of glucose, it cannot grow and multiply and spread. All forms of starch – potatoes, rice, pasta, porridge, bread – are really long chains of glucose molecules, and table sugar is 50 per cent glucose. But more about this in Chapter 5.

Normal cells do not travel around the body and multiply at various locations. In other words, a skin cell remains a skin cell and a liver cell remains in the liver. Cancer cells can travel in the blood vessels or via the lymphatic vessels to other parts of the body and can cause the development of secondary tumours.

The Stages of Cancer

The development of cancer in the body is divided into three main stages. I refer to these as the *seed* stage, the plant stage and the spread stage. Figure 1.2 illustrates the three stages.

The conversion of a normal cell into a cancer cell happens when the DNA, or the genes, of the cell is damaged. This can happen accidentally when cells divide but it can also happen if the body is exposed to radiation, especially ionising radiation such as X-rays, and to certain toxins such as cigarette smoke.

Figure 1.2: *The Three Main Stages of Cancer*

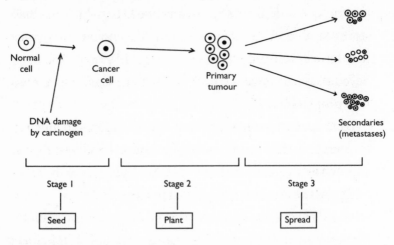

Stage 1 is the process whereby a normal cell converts to a cancer cell. This is the initial stage of cancer formation. Scientists refer to it as **initiation**. I refer to it as the **seed stage** as it resembles the initial stage in the growth of a plant. Without the presence of a *see*d, a plant will not sprout and grow. In this initial stage, the genes that control cell division are damaged, so allowing the cells to divide in an uncontrolled fashion.

For a *see*d to sprout and grow into a plant, it needs water, food and sunlight. These are the things that promote plant development. For a single cancer cell to develop into a primary tumour it needs certain chemicals to promote its growth. These chemicals, or promoters of cancer, have been shown to be certain hormones, such as oestrogen, and certain hormone-like substances called growth factors, such as insulin-like growth factor. Scientists call this stage **promotion**; I refer to it as the **plant stage.**

The third stage of cancer growth involves its spread. Initially the spread is localised and the cancer invades surrounding tissues. Later, the rogue cancer cells can spread to other parts of the body, such as the liver, which has rich stores of glucose. This is very similar to how plants, once they have developed, use insects to spread to other places. I have called this stage the **spread stage** but scientists refer to it as *progression.*

For a cancer to spread, it needs more oxygen and glucose, in essence a rich supply of blood. Local blood vessels can supply the needs of a small tumour, but once it enlarges and grows beyond a certain size – approximately 1 millimetre – it needs to be able to form its own blood vessels to ensure further growth. This ability of malignant tumours to create a network of new blood vessels has significant implications for both the prevention and treatment of cancer.

I mention the above three stages to illustrate the significant points in the development of cancer where different preventive measures can impact its growth. I will return to each stage later in the book, when discussing the various measures that can protect you from developing cancer.

Your Genes Are Only Part of the Picture
Actress Angelina Jolie's decision to have a double mastectomy in 2013 raised the general public's awareness of the role that genes play in the development of cancer. She was advised by her doctors to have the mastectomy as she had a high risk of getting breast cancer based on the fact that she had inherited the now infamous BRCA genes.

However, whether you develop cancer or not is seldom related to your genetic make-up alone. In most cases, it has much more to do with your lifestyle and environment.

DNA is stored in the nucleus of a cell. Scientific research shows that our DNA is wrapped around a group of proteins called histones. These proteins act as a framework to support the DNA, holding it in place. Both the DNA and the protein framework have receptors that receive messages all the time from their environment, that is, the rest of the cell and the rest of the body. These messages have the power to 'switch' genes on or off. In other words, we inherit our genes from both parents but it is the interaction between our genes and their environment that determines whether they are expressed or not.

These receptors on the DNA and its protein framework are called the *epigenomes*. These are a major factor in determining whether you will or will not develop cancer, even if you have inherited the BRCA genes. In the last twenty years, epigenetics has become very important in the field of science and medicine. It shows how all parts of the body are connected and how each cell is aware of what is happening in other parts of the body and even outside the body.

The epigenome constantly changes in response to messages or signals. These signals come from inside the cell, from neighbouring cells, from distant parts of the body and also from the outside world. Each cell is in a constant state of flux as it adjusts to all these signals. In essence, the nucleus of the cell, where the DNA is stored, is the hub of all the activity of the cell. It directs the responses to all the signals received. It is the nerve centre.

By far the single major environmental influence on the epigenome is diet. In your lifetime, diet will play a significant role in determining what diseases you will get. Thus, environment and particularly nutrition play a key role in disease prevention and disease development. When I was at university, it was thought that genes played the major role in cancer development and that cancer was more an inherited disorder than related to diet; nutritional medicine was in its infancy. Epigenetics shows how factors such as diet and stress interact with our genes and the importance of good nutrition and reduced stress in preventive and curative medicine.

Epigenetics has helped us understand better how all the cells of the body are interconnected and how cells respond to their external environment.

WHY THE INCIDENCE OF CANCER HAS INCREASED SINCE 1940

Let us go back now to the reason why cancer has increased so much since the 1940s. Basically, since then we have experienced a huge increase in our exposure to carcinogens, such as chemicals that can initiate cancer and others that can promote the growth and spread of cancer.

The soil, rivers and lakes, and especially the water table have been contaminated with agricultural chemicals. Prior to 1940, farmers did not use nitrogen fertilisers or any chemical sprays on their crops. However, because of the shortage of food during and after the Second World War, farmers were forced by their governments to increase food production using chemical fertiliser.

The problem was that this chemical fertiliser weakened the plants and made them more susceptible to infection. This led to the development of chemical sprays such as pesticides to protect the plants. These pesticides have been used extensively since the 1940s and many younger farmers don't know how to farm without them. The advent of chemical fertilisers and pesticide sprays may have *see*med like a huge advance in agriculture, but in actual fact it has done irreparable damage to our environment and to our health.

Also, since the 1940s, antibiotics have come into widespread use and are now one of the most prescribed drugs worldwide. The overuse or unnecessary use of antibiotics has caused huge damage to the bacterial population that protects each of us, thereby weakening the first line of defence of our immune system. The abuse of antibiotics through over-prescription has led to the development of superbugs, some of which are untreatable. I have dealt with this issue in detail in my book *Antibiotics: Are They Curing Us or Killing Us?*

More and more processed foods have entered the food chain since the 1940s, pushing the natural foods to one side. This has had a hugely negative impact on our immunity. Processed foods contain sugar and white flour, which are known to weaken the immune system, and they are generally deficient in the vitamins, minerals, antioxidants and other important substances that natural foods contain.

Many more hormone disrupters such as plastics and pesticides, not to mention perfumes and other body-care products, have entered the marketplace and are affecting people's health in a profound way, as I will show in Chapter 2.

Then, in the mid-1970s, the food companies reduced the fat in foods, replacing the fat with sugar (*see* Chapter 6). This led to the obesity epidemic and to a further increase in the incidence of cancer.

It is an understatement to say that cancer is a Western disease. It is a direct result of what has gone wrong in

Western society over the past sixty years. Basically, our water supply is no longer safe, our food is weakening us and we have damaged our environment, rendering the planet unsafe from a health perspective. To add fuel to the fire, stress levels have risen sharply over the same period of time. The actions of the food companies and the drug companies, and the inaction of politicians have contributed to the cancer epidemic. But this situation is reversible.

Taking responsibility for our own health is a good start. If we can become more conscious of the dangers in our everyday environment, adjust our diet to a natural one rich in anti-cancer foods and reduce our stress levels then we are perfectly capable of avoiding cancer completely.

SUMMARY

Every one of us develops cancer cells every day in our bodies because of small errors as cells divide and multiply. Every day our immune cells, especially natural killer cells, take care of these abnormal cells by destroying them. They are the special forces of the immune system.

Carcinogens are substances or radiation in our food or our environment that are able to damage our DNA and so initiate cancer. Carcinogens are the *see*ds that can grow into cancer. Exposure to carcinogens is not the factor that will determine if you get cancer; rather, your immune system will determine that, as the case of Mighty Mouse showed.

Prior to 1940 there were low levels of cancer but since then cancer has become an epidemic in the Western world. This is mainly the result of environmental pollution and dietary changes.

Chapter 2
Your Environment

Case History – Jane

Jane was a 35-year-old woman who came to seek my help with ongoing digestive issues. She was a very aware person in that she was eating an excellent diet and was familiar with a lot of the issues I deal with in this book. She told me that she lived on a street in Dublin of about thirty houses and that no fewer than seven of the families on the street had lost a loved one to cancer. She herself had had bowel cancer and had part of her colon removed.

She also told me that every time she went on holidays or was away from home for a period of time, she began to feel more energetic and was generally in better form. Many of her neighbours also reported the same experience. When I questioned her further, it transpired that there was an electricity substation at the end of her street.

I suggested that she move back to her parents' house, which wasn't far away, and that she have her house tested for electromagnetic disturbances. The results of these tests indicated that there was a very strong electrical field emanating from the substation – Jane's house was the third closest to the substation.

I'm not sure what happened after this. Much later, I heard from one of her friends that she had taken the electricity company to court but that the case was ongoing.

This is one of numerous stories that I have heard over the years concerning electrical pylons, underground cables and substations. In many countries it is against the law to build a house within 500 metres of an electrical overhead cable or substation. However, it is not against the law in much of Europe, including Ireland and the UK.

The IARC considers the electrical fields generated by overhead and underground cables, as well as substations, to be a possible cause of human cancer. It appears that the closer you live to the cable or substation, the greater your risk of developing the disease (IARC, 1995). The key statement that Jane made, which alarmed me, was that she felt better when she left home for a period of time. If you feel ill in one location and improve on moving away to another location, this is highly suggestive of a problem with the first location. In this circumstance, the reasons why one might feel ill can vary, but one of the most common reasons relates to the land on which your house is built.

In addition to electromagnetic energy generated by pylons and substations, there are a range of chemicals in our environment that can also explain the huge rise in the incidence of cancer. The most prevalent and arguably the most significant chemicals, as regards causing cancer, are those that act on the hormonal system; they are referred to as hormone disrupters. Let's examine these in detail as they are thought to be responsible for the huge increase in hormonal cancers, such as breast cancer in women and prostate cancer in men (IARC, 1995).

OESTROGEN AND OTHER HORMONE DISRUPTERS IN YOUR ENVIRONMENT

I feel that it is important for you to become aware of the environmental sources of oestrogen and other hormone disrupters, so that you can avoid them and teach your children to avoid them. The following is a list of the main culprits, though there are many others.

Pesticides

I mentioned pesticides in Chapter 1, and my book *Good Food: Can You Trust What You Are Eating?* also covers them in detail.

These chemicals are used to kill plant-eating insects and fungi. For obvious reasons, the workers in the factories where these chemicals are made and the farmers who spray them on their crops have the highest levels of exposure.

However, because these chemicals remain in the environment for years and can be leached by rain water into the water table below, anyone who drinks well water may be at risk. These chemicals have also shown up in breads and cereals, which implies widespread exposure.

These same chemicals are also used on textiles and can enter your home in blankets, sofas, beds, carpets and other household items. They are used to kill household pests such as cockroaches, flies and wasps. They are also used in tick and lice treatments for humans and for pets. In addition, they are used across the world as mosquito repellents and to kill mosquitoes.

The most famous, or should I say infamous, pesticide is undoubtedly DDT, which, although banned for years, still shows up as present in the environment. This pesticide can remain in the environment for decades, still doing harm, and it routinely shows up in the fat tissue of birds and other animals.

It is high time all pesticides were banned, if we are serious about tackling the true causes of cancer.

Buy only organic fruit; if you can't do this, only eat fruit that you can peel, such as oranges, lemons and bananas. Reduce or avoid commercial cereals in your diet or buy organic cereals instead. Try to buy organic meat. Avoid all processed meats such as cold ham, turkey, salami and pepperoni.

Plastics

Different kinds of plastics are found everywhere in the home; food is bought and stored in plastic containers. However, dangerous chemicals are used to make plastics. For years it was thought that plastics were indestructible and so did not break down if left exposed. Scientists have now discovered that much of the plastic waste floating in the world's oceans not only breaks down but does so quite rapidly. These plastics are reduced to the original chemicals used to make them and these chemicals in turn pollute the environment in which they are found. If plastic decays in the ocean, the chemicals will harm the fish. If you thought wild Atlantic fish was safe, you'd better adjust your thinking.

In the home, plastics are found in bottles, bowls, storage containers, kettles and children's toys. A major study looking at the risk to human health from household plastics found that over 30 per cent of these plastics leached dangerous chemicals into the surrounding environment (Muncke, 2011).

When I was growing up in the 1950s and 1960s, all liquids such as milk or lemonade came in glass bottles. Nowadays, it's hard to find any liquid or food that comes in glass containers. Another research study showed that spring water in plastic bottles had three times the oestrogenic activity of the same water in glass bottles (Wagner, 2011). This is definitive proof that these hormone-disrupting chemicals are finding their way into our food and drink.

In the absence of an all-out ban on all forms of plastic in our environment, we must start the process in our own homes. Here is a list of suggestions:

- Remove all plastic kettles, cutlery, bowls, plates, etc.
- Do not feed your baby from a plastic bottle.
- Buy your food and drink in glass containers.
- Remove all children's plastic toys.
- Do not store any food in plastic wrap or a plastic container; transfer to paper or foil.
- If you have pvc pipes, have them replaced when you can afford it.

Drugs

Back in the 1980s there was a very interesting report published in various magazines and newspapers about the meat market in Paris. In the market there are strong macho guys that carry the carcasses for the butchers. These macho men are referred to as *les forts*, which translates as 'the strong ones'. They are very proud of their masculinity.

When, to their embarrassment, these macho men began to grow breast tissue, there was an investigation to discover why. The butchers used to make a delicacy for these men using the necks of chickens. When the investigators traced the source of these chickens, they discovered that their necks were being injected with stilbestrol, a synthetic form of oestrogen used to increase the size of the bird (oestrogen increases body weight). This is an example of how drugs can find their way into the human food chain, causing hormonal problems.

The contraceptive pill, hormone replacement therapy, cimetidine to treat peptic ulcers and diethylstilbestrol are all hormone disrupters that millions of people around the world use on a daily basis. When excreted from the body as urine, they enter the water system. In many cities and towns around the world this waste water is pumped to a water treatment plant where it is recycled and returned as tap water. Since oestrogen is hard to remove, much of the oestrogen remains in the water after treatment and enters your home in the tap water.

For this reason, I would strongly urge against the use of tap water for drinking, making tea or cooking. It is safe to use tap water to wash or brush teeth provided you don't swallow any of it. Tap water is unhealthy because it may contain oestrogen, chlorine and fluorine, as well as heavy metals such as lead, cadmium and arsenic. I discuss this in more detail in Chapter 3.

A reverse osmosis purifier can remove many of the chemicals from tap water, but even with this you cannot guarantee the removal of oestrogen.

Heavy Metals
There are a number of metals that can disrupt the hormonal system, among them arsenic and cadmium.

The IARC classifies substances based on their potential to cause cancer. Category 1 substances are definitely carcinogenic. Arsenic and cadmium fall into this category.

Arsenic
This metal usually accumulates in the soil and water table where there has been a history of mining and smelting. Parts of Devon and Cornwall in the UK have particularly high levels of arsenic as a result of mining activity. In fact, during the 1800s Cornwall was the world's largest producer of arsenic. Arsenic is used in a number of industrial activities, such as manufacturing car batteries, smelting copper and lead, and as a wood preservative. It is also used in the manufacture of pesticides used in agriculture.

In parts of the world where there are high levels of arsenic in the soil, such as in some of the rice-growing areas of India, Bangladesh, Thailand and China, this metal can leak into the water table and then enter the plants. When it enters plants that we eat, such as rice, the metal can enter the food chain and cause illness and, in some cases, death. The highest incidence of cancer caused by arsenic is in Bangladesh.

As you may already be aware from detective novels and murder mystery programmes, ingesting high levels of arsenic can cause death. Exposure to low levels over a period of time can irritate the gut, causing nausea, vomiting and diarrhoea, as well as causing areas of darker pigmentation or patches of depigmentation on the skin. Later it causes thickening of the skin, warts and, later still, skin cancer. The gut and skin symptoms are usually what the patient presents with, but arsenic is known to affect a number of organs. It can affect the hormonal system, causing diabetes; it can affect the bone marrow, causing anaemia; it can affect the nervous system, causing peripheral neuropathy; it can affect the kidneys, causing blood or glucose in the urine; and it can cause cardiac arrhythmia or irregular heartbeat.

Arsenic appears to be even more toxic to children. It has been implicated in causing a lower IQ in children. Because arsenic can cross the placenta it may cause harm to an unborn baby. Studies carried out on laboratory animals would appear to substantiate this, as these have shown arsenic to cause low birth weight, malformation and even death (Ferm, 1977).

To reduce your risk of exposure to arsenic, avoid tap water, especially in areas with high arsenic levels in the soil or water table. If in doubt, ask your county council or a private water-testing company to check your tap water or well water for metals. Wood is often treated with arsenic. Avoid exposure to sawdust, especially if you are a carpenter or involved in DIY projects at home. Avoid rice products imported from parts of the world that are known to have high levels of arsenic in the soil.

Cadmium

The detrimental effects of this metal on human health are demonstrated by the story of a strange illness that affected people in one particular region of Japan, Toyama Prefecture, from the early twentieth century. This strange illness was given the name '*itai-itai* disease', which translates into English as 'it hurts-it hurts disease'.

Since the early 1900s people in Toyama Prefecture suffered from a range of symptoms, including severe joint and bone pain – hence 'it hurts-it hurts' – brittle bones and kidney problems. They blamed the local mining company, Mitsui Mining and Smelting Co. Ltd, for polluting the river and thus poisoning the fish and plants that were their main sources of food; even the rice fields were irrigated using the water from the river.

It was not until the 1960s that the mining company was forced by the courts to compensate those who had suffered from '*itai-itai* disease', including the relatives of locals who had died of the disease. It was proved in court that the mining company had contaminated the river with high levels of cadmium, which is a metal that is known to cause these symptoms. This case in Japan is often cited to explain some of the most noticeable symptoms of cadmium toxicity and to identify the possible sources of cadmium exposure.

In the West, by far the most common source of exposure to this metal is cigarette smoke. This is the main reason why the smoking ban was introduced in certain countries. In comparison to nonsmokers, smokers are found to have much higher levels of cadmium in their blood and kidneys. Passive smokers are also at risk of developing cadmium toxicity.

Other people at risk of cadmium exposure include those working in the mining or smelting of metals, those working in the manufacturing of batteries, especially cadmium-nickel batteries, and also those who come into contact with contaminated food or water, as in Japan.

As we *see* with the case in Japan, the effects of cadmium exposure on the human body are severe bone and joint pain as well as osteoporosis and kidney problems. In fact, the kidney is the main target organ for cadmium as the metal binds to kidney tissues and damages them. Other symptoms include fatigue, dry skin and yellow teeth.

Cadmium exposure can also affect our hormonal system, and this is where it is particularly relevant to our discussion of cancer. In male workers who have had significant occupational exposure to cadmium – such as those working in the mining, smelting or battery manufacturing industries – there is evidence of altered levels of male sex hormones. Some of these workers have also suffered damage to and ultimately cancer of the prostate and testes. In 1993, the IARC classified cadmium as a definite carcinogen on the basis of a review of all the scientific data available at that time.

Other Metals in Our Environment
In September 2014, Irish Water was reported as saying that approximately 10 per cent of water supplies in Ireland have excessive levels of lead (Melia, 2014). That means one in ten homes is being exposed to lead through the water supply. This does not take into account the excessive levels of other metals such as arsenic, cadmium and aluminium in our tap water. Tap water is clearly not fit for human consumption.

Dentists in Ireland and the UK are still using dental amalgams, another major source of metal exposure. If a person with metal fillings clenches or grinds their teeth, they can wear away the metal. Particles of the metal fillings can enter the saliva, be swallowed into the gut and be absorbed into the body, where they can lodge and cause a range of problems.

Amalgam fillings are made up of 50 per cent mercury and 25 per cent silver; the remaining 25 per cent is a mixture of other metals. Dentists who don't use metal fillings claim that all mercury fillings continuously release a vapour that can be breathed in and cause toxicity. If you wish to have your metal fillings replaced, go to an amalgam-free dental practice as the dentists are trained to protect you when removing the fillings.

In truth, because of the prevalence of metals in our environment, it is really important to get tested for the presence of metals in your system and, if they are present, remove them or the sources of them. Metals are a very powerful block to healing and are toxic to the body, especially mercury and lead. The metals which are carcinogenic include arsenic, chromium and cadmium. To prevent cancer, make sure you get tested for these metals in particular. The simplest mode of testing is to carry out a 6-hour or a 24-hour urine collection and have it tested for a range of toxic metals. I do this for many of my patients because I have *seen* how beneficial it can be for people, and it has been enormously helpful in my own life.

Perfumes, Deodorants and Cosmetics

You may be surprised to read that many of the common products for sale to beautify your body and make you smell good are full of chemicals that not only disrupt the hormonal system but have been implicated in hormonal cancers such as breast cancer.

All of these personal care products are made from synthetic chemicals. There is mounting evidence that not only are the individual chemicals harmful to humans but the mixture of chemicals may be especially harmful. This harm is most pronounced at critical periods of human development, such as the prenatal stage, the early years of life and puberty.

The UK-based group Campaign for Safe Cosmetics recently tested a number of the top-selling brands of perfumes for men and women. They found a range of hormone-disrupting chemicals in them. Worse still, they also found a number of allergens that were not identified on the labels but which are known to cause asthma, contact dermatitis and headaches. Some of the big-name brands contained as many as twelve hormone disrupters, some of which are known to mimic oestrogen and to be involved in the growth and development of breast cancer (Campaign for Safe Cosmetics and Environmental Working Group, 2010).

Citral was one of the chemicals identified. This is a very common ingredient in perfumes and is known to cause prostate enlargement in laboratory animals. It has also been shown to have oestrogenic effects in the same animals. It is a true hormone disrupter.

Parabens are a group of chemicals present in almost all personal care products and even in some food items. All of these chemicals interfere with hormone levels in the body and all have been shown to be capable of mimicking oestrogen.

There is a general belief that these perfumes are quite safe to use and many people use them frequently. This belief is based on the trust that it would be made public if these products were harmful in any way. The truth is that the cosmetic and perfume industries are critical to the economy of many countries and are worth billions every year – the cosmetics industry was worth €58.79 billion in the USA in 2014, for example (www.statista.com/statistics/243742/revenue-of-the-cosmetic-industry-in-the-us). No wonder many of the top celebrities advertise toiletries and cosmetics to boost their income. Many harmful ingredients do not need to be declared as the cosmetics and perfume industries claim that it would damage their advantage over competitors to disclose the composition of their products. As a consequence, products containing harmful ingredients can be sold to the public without any regulation.

Clearly, this needs to change. Public awareness campaigns as to the dangers lurking in beauty products should be more widespread and celebrities should choose whether to join such campaigns or continue to promote hormone-damaging chemicals and carcinogens. Strict warnings should also be applied to these products and much more research needs to be done to ascertain the extent of the damage they can cause.

In the interim, I would advise being very cautious in the use of such products.

I would suggest that you only buy products that use safe substances in the manufacturing process. Some companies only use only plant-based ingredients in the production of make-up and toiletries, thus avoiding harmful chemicals such as parabens. One such company is the Organic Pharmacy (www.theorganicpharmacy.com), but there are actually a growing number of these companies selling safer, more ethical products.

———

In the 1920s and 1930s, doctors and scientists first became aware of the potential risk posed by synthetic chemicals in the Western world. At that time doctors such as Sir Robert

McCarrison had declared the Hunza people of West Pakistan and the Sikh population of India as cancer free. In fact, many isolated peoples were then cancer free. These scientists and doctors began to link the rise of the chemical industry in certain parts of the world with the increased incidence of cancer in these areas.

Then in the 1960s, with the publication of Rachel Carson's book *Silent Spring*, the public became more aware of the risks posed by agricultural chemicals in particular. Today there are thousands of chemicals in the environment, many of which have not been tested for safety; in truth, we know little about some of these and what damage they can cause, especially when they are used in the combinations we find in the products we use in our homes. These chemicals are known to accumulate in living creatures and are concentrated in the bodies of animals high up the food chain.

Today, the polar bear is one of the most polluted animals on the planet. This might *seem* strange, considering that these animals live far from human habitation. However, it has become apparent to scientists that pollutants in the sea that are ingested by smaller fish become more concentrated in the larger fish that eat them. These bigger fish, such as salmon and sea trout, are then eaten by bears, who over time accumulate even higher levels of these chemicals, making them a highly polluted species. But not the most polluted.

That position is reserved for the animal at the top of the food chain, the animal that grows and manufactures its own food, the animal that pollutes the rest of creation – humans. We are the most toxic species alive and we are entirely responsible for compromising the health of other species, including the polar bear.

IONISING RADIATION

As well as electromagnetic energy and hormone disrupters, harmful amounts of ionising radiation in our environment can threaten our health and lead to cancer. Ionising radiation is a form of radiation that can penetrate the body and damage our genetic material or DNA. When DNA is damaged there is the potential for cancer to develop. Ionising radiation can therefore be regarded as an initiator of cancer; it can form the *seed* for cancer to develop.

There are many forms of ionising radiation, the most common of which is X-rays. When X-rays were first developed they were used by shop assistants in shoe shops to accurately measure foot size but then the hazards of X-ray exposure became apparent and the practice stopped. Other forms of ionising radiation are used in CAT scans and PET scans to assist with medical diagnosis.

Let's look at the more common forms of ionising radiation in our environment.

Radon Gas

Where there is uranium in the soil, radon gas can be formed, as it is a breakdown product of uranium. Being a gas, it can *seep* into homes and workspaces from the underlying soil. It is known to cause lung cancer (Gray *et al.*, 2009). The danger lies in the fact that radon gas is difficult to detect as it is invisible and odourless.

Exposure to radon gas is far from a minor problem as it is the second leading cause of cancer deaths in the USA, killing more than 21,000 people annually (www.epa.gov/radon/pubs/citguide.html). In the UK, the level of radon in the soil is generally lower and so the number of deaths attributable to the gas is lower.

Because radon gas is formed from the radioactive decay of uranium, it is classified as a major source of ionising radiation, along with X-rays and CAT scans. Chronic exposure to any form of ionising radiation significantly increases the risk of cancer.

If you live or work in an area where there is a lot of granite or limestone rock, it is worth your while getting your home or office checked. Contact your local branch of the Environment Protection Agency (EPA) (or equivalent) and they will supply you with a kit for checking the levels of radon gas and all the necessary information (*see* www.epa. ie/radiation).

Other Forms of Ionising Radiation

Radon accounts for about 50 per cent of our exposure to dangerous ionising radiation. Medical procedures account for another 20 per cent approximately, but this varies from country to country and depends mainly on how frequently doctors advise patients to have procedures that can result in exposure.

Two medical procedures that can result in exposure to ionising radiation are CAT scans and X-rays, especially the former. To put it into perspective, almost 2,000 patients contract cancer every year in the UK because of medical diagnostic procedures (Djamgoz and Plant, 2014). This figure is much higher in other countries, such as the USA where doctors are much quicker to suggest CAT scans. The number of CAT scans in the USA has increased markedly over the recent past – from 3 million in 1980 to 62 million in 2006 (NCRP, 2009).

There is much concern both inside and outside the medical profession about the widespread use of CAT scans. Basically, a CAT scan uses a dose of radiation 500 to 1,000 times greater than that used in a normal chest X-ray. Therefore, to protect patients, many of whom are not aware of this fact, CAT scans should be reserved for exceptional situations and the risks should be explained to the patient. There is particular concern in the medical profession about the use of CAT scans on children.

Because of the higher risk of cancer associated with CAT scans, if your doctor suggests a CAT scan ask him or her for an alternative investigation such as ultrasound or even an MRI scan. If you are in the radiology department and about to have a diagnostic procedure performed, always ask to have the risks explained to you. In other words, you must make an informed decision. If you do not have sufficient information or are in doubt, perhaps delay the procedure.

NON-IONISING RADIATION
Non-ionising radiation is less penetrative of human tissue and therefore thought to be less harmful. In general, it does not appear to damage DNA and so initiate cancer. Non-ionising radiation is emitted by mobile phones. However, there is now growing concern that keeping a mobile phone close to your body for lengthy periods of time or living close to a mobile phone mast or tower may have health risks.

Mobile Phones and Masts

The IARC suggests that the radiation given off by mobile phones and by the masts that supply signal is a possible carcinogen. Early studies suggested that there was little or no risk, but more recent research suggests a possible link between this radiation and brain cancers (Hardell, 2009). So living close to a mobile phone mast or frequent use of a mobile phone may indeed increase your risk of getting cancer.

Having said that, other evidence suggests that mobile phones and masts are relatively safe (Yakyemenko and Sidorik, 2010). More research is definitely needed as phone usage has increased considerably over the past twenty years and many children now carry mobile phones.

A large study of mobile phone use and possible effects on health has been under way in Europe since 2010. This study, known as Cosmos, will follow almost 300,000 adults over a twenty-year period, so its results will not be known for many years.

It is thought that children are at greater risk than adults of developing brain cancers from mobile phones. This is based on the fact that the nervous system of children is still developing and is therefore more susceptible to disruption.

Until the debate about mobile phone safety has been decided, it is advisable to follow the path of maximum safety for you and your family. Here are a few guidelines.

- Keep mobile phones and routers as far away from your body as possible.
- When talking on a mobile phone, use a hands-free set or switch sides (left ear to right ear) frequently.

- Keep mobile phones away from children.
- Limit the amount of time you are on a mobile phone; use a landline if you have to make lots of calls.
- Turn off the mobile phone before you sleep at night or else keep the device far away from your body, especially your head.

SUMMARY

Many of us are exposed to different forms of radiation. Some of these forms of radiation are known to be very damaging to the body, especially to our genes or DNA. These include CAT and PET scans, X-rays and the breakdown of radioactive elements in the soil, such as uranium, to radon gas.

There are other forms of radiation that are presently thought to be safer, such as non-ionising radiation from MRI scans, mobile phones and mobile phone masts or towers. However, recent research would advise caution in the use of these devices.

If you are concerned that your home is located too close to a mobile phone mast, contact your local branch of the EPA and they will measure the level of radiation and advise you further.

Chapter 3
What You Put into Your Body

This chapter deals with what I regard as the most important cancer prevention tools at your disposal – the food and drink you consume on a daily basis.

One of the reasons why cancer is so uncommon among isolated peoples such as the Inuit is that such people are completely dependent on nature and do not *see* themselves as separate from it. Their food and drink are almost 100 per cent natural and their bodies are in sync with the natural cycle.

In contrast, we in the West have become separated from nature and are out of sync with the natural order. We try to manipulate nature to suit our own ends. Nowhere is this more apparent than in the manufacturing of our own food. Our homes are full of tins, bottles, jars and packets, and we consume large quantities of microwave meals, TV dinners, takeaways and so on. This is where the disconnection between nature and those leading a Western lifestyle starts to have a serious impact on health. We *see* the major difference between city dwellers and isolated peoples in what they consume on a daily basis.

To avoid cancer and remain healthy, we have to realise that our bodies need certain substances that can only be supplied by natural foods. This requires a shift in our thinking – do not rely on your supermarket for food; rather, look around for other sources of food, such as local farmers' markets. Nature has a vested interest in keeping you well, whereas the wider food industry doesn't care a hoot about your well-being.

There are a number of problems concerning what we Westerners eat and drink. I will show how these are contributing to the rise in cancer. First, let's examine what we drink.

WATER

There is a common misconception that our bodies are 90 per cent water. For many years in my practice, I have used a computerised device called a Body Composition Analyser, which analyses the body to indicate its levels of water, fat, protein and so on. The truth is that most people's bodies are composed of between 50 and 60 per cent water. Men have a bit more than women. Children's bodies have higher water content – anything up to 75 per cent.

The interior of a cell is mostly water, these cells are surrounded by tissue fluid, which is water, and the blood that circulates around your body is mainly composed of water. More than half your body is water and therefore water forms the single most important part of your diet. The water you are consuming is the first thing to become aware of if you are serious about avoiding cancer.

The quality of your drinking water dictates how efficiently your body functions. The purer the water, the easier it is for your body to use it. The purity of drinking water has become a major issue in many countries and people have become more alert to what is being added to their tap water.

The Problems with Tap Water

Fluoride

The element fluorine is essential for good health. It is needed to strengthen bones, teeth, nails and hair. It even strengthens tendons. It does this by combining with calcium to form the compound calcium fluoride. Raw fruit and vegetables are natural sources of fluoride. If the vegetable or fruit is heated, boiled or steamed, the fluoride is destroyed. To ensure maximum levels of fluoride in your body, you should allow raw foods to become an essential part of your diet. Foods especially rich in fluorine include sea vegetables, avocados, black-eyed peas, cabbage, cauliflower, Brussels sprouts and all green vegetables, such as spinach.

However, this element has many other functions in the body. It is often referred to as an anti-ageing substance. Found in the elastic tissue of skin, it strengthens skin sufficiently to delay the onset of wrinkles, which form due to a loss of elasticity. It is also anti-ageing in that it maintains the structural integrity of bones and teeth, thus reducing the leaching of calcium from these structures with age. If you wish to prevent osteoporosis, ensure you have adequate levels of fluorine in your system by eating lots of uncooked vegetables and fruit.

Fluorine has a very positive effect on the immune system as well. It is important for the smooth functioning of the spleen. The spleen, which sits under your left ribcage, is part of the lymphatic system and is therefore important in strengthening your immunity. Fluorine protects you against harmful bacteria and viruses.

You may well ask why I am writing about the benefits of fluorine when this chapter should be concerned with its harmful effects. I want you to be aware of the beneficial form of fluorine before discussing the harmful form. The beneficial form, as I mentioned above, is *calcium fluoride*. However, this is not what is added to tap water in some countries.

The compound that is added to tap water is *sodium fluoride*, a completely different substance. According to the Merck Index, it is a rat and cockroach poison. Admittedly, it is used in very low levels in drinking water, with the aim of reducing dental cavities. The argument is that the level is low enough to be safe. This is the same argument presented by the authorities for the many harmful chemicals that are added to processed foods and drinks. My argument is that the issue is not one of short-term safety but rather one of long-term toxicity. There is enough evidence to ban sodium fluoride now, especially since most toothpaste has fluoride in it, thereby making the addition of sodium fluoride to water totally unnecessary.

The fluoridation of water is achieved by adding chemicals that contain fluoride to it, such as sodium fluoride in the USA or hydrofluorosilicic acid in Ireland. The former is a by-product of an industrial process, while the latter is a by-product of the manufacture of fertilisers. Both are industrial waste products and both are toxic.

It is common knowledge now that fluoride causes damage to bones and teeth. It combines with calcium and magnesium in bones and weakens their structure, resulting in osteoporosis in adults and rickets in children. It discolours the teeth in addition to weakening them. However, it does much more than this if you are exposed to it long term.

Chlorine

Chlorine is added to tap water to kill any bad bugs that may be present in the water. This is the same reason why chlorine is added to swimming-pool water.

It is not a bad intention. However, chlorine kills all bacteria, including the good bacteria that protect your body and your gut in particular. Taking into account the very important role of the bacterial population of the body in the health of the immune system, we should avoid chlorine as much as possible.

Metals

There are a number of metals in our water supply that are classified as carcinogenic by the IARC. Such metals include arsenic, cadmium, chromium and nickel. Recent reports from the IARC classify lead as a probable carcinogen based on animal and human studies (www.iarc.fr).

On 19 September 2014, a headline appeared on the front page of the *Irish Independent* newspaper: 'One in ten homes at risk from lead in water'. The article states that, since many of the old lead pipes have not been replaced in many areas of the country, 10 per cent of Irish homes are at risk of lead poisoning due to ageing pipes.

Lead is highly toxic to humans, which is the reason why it has been removed from petrol, paint and solder. In many countries lead pipes have been replaced with plastic or copper pipes, but in many cities, including Dublin and London, there are still lead pipes under the streets and in some old houses. When taking a medical history from my patients, I always ask about their water supply and about possible exposure to lead in particular. If an individual lived in a city before lead was removed from petrol, this is significant as he or she may have been breathing in lead in exhaust fumes. Also, if the house a person lives in is old or he or she went to an old boarding school, then that information may be helpful. If I am suspicious of metal toxicity from a person's history or from the symptoms that he or she presents with, I will test that person for a range of metals. Table 3.1 lists the common symptoms associated with having a high level of lead in your system:

Table 3.1: Symptoms of Lead Toxicity

Anaemia

Anorexia

Anxiety

Concentration impairment

Confusion

Constipation

Depression

Dizziness

Drowsiness

Fatigue

Headache

Hypertension

Indigestion

Irritability

Lack of coordination

Memory impairment

Pain in abdomen

Pain in bones

Pain in muscles

Restlessness

Tremors

I am very familiar with some of these symptoms because I have had them since childhood. I grew up in the countryside and we had our own well dug in our back garden. The water from this well was pumped through to our house via lead pipes and as a result I ended up with lead in my body. After years of treating others for lead poisoning, it dawned on me that I might also have the same problem. I tested myself and discovered I had a number of metals at toxic levels in my system, including mercury and nickel.

Another metal that is found in tap water and is definitely carcinogenic is arsenic. I discuss the effects of arsenic on our health in Chapter 2. In Bangladesh, 20 per cent of deaths every year are attributed to the toxic effects of arsenic in food and water. Certain cancers associated with arsenic are therefore very common in that part of the world, most notably skin cancer, liver cancer and bladder cancer.

The Institute for Food Safety in Queen's University, Belfast recently discovered that there was arsenic in the food chain, and they detected high levels of this metal in rice products. Professor Andy Meharg tested many food samples containing rice, including a number of baby foods, and was alarmed by what he found. He reported his findings to the Food Standards Agency in the UK. He quickly became aware that there were no controls in place to restrict foods with high levels of arsenic, even though it is widely known that this metal is poisonous (Sommella *et al.*, 2013).

Dr Diane Bedford of the Food Standards Agency in London has said that she is waiting for guidelines from the WHO before acting (Sommella *et al.*, 2013). Using delay tactics in an effort to protect the food manufacturers is the way the Food Standards Agency in the UK and the European

Food Safety Authority *seem* to operate. They are political bodies controlled by politicians and can therefore be subject to interference by food manufacturers and drug companies.

In the light of this important information, it is wise to restrict rice-based foods in your diet, including rice milk and baby cereals containing rice, not to mention plain rice itself. It *seem*s as though foods that were once safe to eat are progressively becoming subject to the effects of pollutants. It is time for the authorities to act and stop the destruction of the whole food chain.

———

My honest advice is not to wait for government agencies to protect you and your family. Rather, take it into your own hands to avoid tap water. I discuss testing the purity of your tap water and alternatives to tap water in Chapter 6.

I shall now discuss some of the foods linked with cancer, both in terms of promotion and prevention.

FOODS LINKED WITH CANCER
High Glycaemic Index Foods
Glycaemic index (GI) is a number that describes the level to which a particular food affects blood glucose level. Water, for example, would have no effect on blood glucose and so its GI is zero on a scale of one to one hundred. Pure glucose, on the other hand, would raise blood glucose to a maximum and so would have a GI of one hundred on this scale.

It is now known that foods with a high GI, such as table sugar and wheat, increase your risk of cancer. I shall discuss sugar and wheat in more detail in Chapter 5, but for the moment I want to highlight them as foods that have a high GI. Such foods increase your risk of cancer by making more glucose available to cancer cells, which use the sugar to multiply. Effectively, it's a bit like throwing petrol on a burning building; you are promoting the growth and spread of the fire.

These foods also promote the growth of cancer in another way. When you eat sugar, for example, your blood glucose levels rise sharply. This in turn stimulates the release of insulin, which pushes the glucose into all cells, including cancer cells. However, a rise in blood glucose levels also stimulates the release of a substance called insulin-like growth factor, abbreviated to IGF, which is known to stimulate cell growth and division. It is one of a number of growth factors that are heavily implicated in the growth and spread of cancer.

As I mentioned in Chapter 1, the intake of high GI foods such as sugar and flour has skyrocketed since the Second World War. This is part of the reason why cancer has increased markedly in the last sixty years. Sugar consumption rose from 2 kilograms per person per year in 1800 to 70 kilograms per person per year in 2004 (Servan-Schreiber, 2011). This staggering increase was due to the rise of the sugar industry, from the increased number of sugar plantations in North and South America and in the Caribbean, to the increase in the number of food manufacturers who added sugar to their food in order to sell it.

As mentioned in Chapter 1, during and after the Second World War the consumption of cheap foods made with sugar and flour increased and, in line with this, the incidence of various cancers increased too. Then in 1974 the major food companies decided to reduce or remove fat from their products and used sugar to replace it. This may be the reason why breast cancer incidence shows a second peak in the mid-seventies.

IGF doesn't only promote the growth and spread of cancer. Science has shown that it reduces the effectiveness of chemotherapy. In laboratory mice, breast cancer cells are less responsive to various anti-cancer drugs (chemotherapy) when the diet is rich in sugar. This discovery has led to a search for drugs that block the release of IGF. But wouldn't it be easier to reduce our intake of foods with a high glycaemic index and replace them with low-glycaemic foods? I will discuss IGF further in Chapter 5.

High-GI foods include all forms of sugar, syrups, white flour, white rice and white pasta, breakfast cereals, jams and marmalades, sweetened drinks and potatoes. For a full list, go to Table 5.1 in Chapter 5.

It would be wise to reduce the high-GI foods in your diet to a minimum and only eat them on rare occasions. Alternatively, avoid them completely. Instead of breakfast cereals, use oats, quinoa or spelt muesli. Use spelt bread or spelt pasta as alternatives to ordinary bread and pasta. Good natural sweeteners are stevia and xylitol.

Dairy Produce

I grew up in the countryside surrounded by farms. As a family, we used to drink raw milk fresh from the cow. It was only when I went to school that I began drinking pasteurised milk. Today, virtually all milk available is pasteurised.

There is now definitive evidence that the main protein in milk, casein, is a promoter of cancer. The bulk of the scientific research was carried out by Professor Campbell of Cornell University in the USA (Campbell and Campbell, 2006). The evidence is so convincing that many countries are now altering their food pyramids or food plates to exclude dairy. Harvard Public Health Laboratory has removed dairy products from its food plate, which is a healthy eating plan used to promote a healthy diet (www.hsph.harvard.edu/nutritionsource/what-should-you-eat/pyramid). This move, based on the latest science, shows an interesting development in the thinking of an institution that has been for so long compromised by its association with the major food companies in the USA.

I believe that it is not dairy that is the problem but rather the process of pasteurisation. During this process, the milk is subjected to high temperatures to kill all the bacteria. High temperatures are known to alter the structure of proteins in the milk and may render them toxic.

If dairy were a problem, the Maasai in East Africa and the Fulani in West Africa, both of whom herd cattle and depend on a supply of milk every day as their main source of food, would show evidence of a high incidence of cancer; but their incidence of cancer is close to zero. Therefore, Professor Campbell is incorrect to blame dairy produce; rather, it's human interference with the production of milk.

You should reduce or avoid pasteurised milk in your diet. Instead, favour soya milk, raw goat's or sheep's milk, or find out where you can buy raw milk directly from a farmer.

I shall discuss dairy further in Chapter 5.

Oils

In the past, foods used to have an equal amount of omega 6 and omega 3 fatty acids. When I was growing up, hens used to be fed on natural forage, not cereals. As a consequence, the hens produced eggs that were rich in omega 3 as well as omega 6. The ratio of omega 6 to omega 3 was 1:1, meaning that the two existed in equal quantities. Today, hens' eggs have very low levels of omega 3 because of the way hens are being fed.

It is necessary to eat foods rich in omega 3 if you wish to avoid cancer. These foods are flaxseed oil and fish oil. Use ground flaxseeds on food or take adequate levels of fish oil every day. Omega 3 is your best friend when it comes to protecting you.

I recommend flaxseed, either as milled seeds or as oil, to all my patients. Because it is also a bulking agent, I use it in treating gut problems as it helps to regularise the bowel habit. It also has the added advantage of reducing inflammation in the gut. I discuss omega 3 and 6 oils further in Chapter 5.

CHRONIC INFLAMMATION AND CANCER

Chronic inflammation is now known to be a major risk factor in the development of cancer. The next case history illustrates this.

Years ago while working in Africa, I remember one particular patient who was admitted to the hospital with skin cancer. This was a very unusual case of malignant melanoma because the patient was a black man. I was taught that melanoma was found mainly in light-skinned people and was a consequence of exposure to sunlight. Melanoma did not occur in Africans as their skin was protected from ultraviolet radiation from the sun by high levels of melanin, the substance that makes their skin dark. Yet here in front of me was an African man with diagnosed melanoma on his foot.

Our pathologist explained that melanoma was possible in the African population in areas of skin where there was chronic inflammation. Sure enough, this man had precisely that – he had a chronic wound on his foot that hadn't healed and was subject to abrasion daily as he walked everywhere barefoot. This was a powerful example of how chronic inflammation can result in cancer.

Inflammation is a normal healthy process and is the means by which your body heals itself. If you cut yourself, the wound quickly becomes red, hot and sore – it becomes inflamed. White blood cells are drawn into the area, as are platelets. These release very important chemicals called inflammatory factors, which guide the process of repair.

Cancer cells need lots of inflammatory factors to stimulate cell division, create new blood vessels for their supply of glucose and allow for the invasion of neighbouring tissues. The University of Glasgow has done a lot of research on these inflammatory factors, which has shown that the levels of inflammatory factors in the body can be used to predict a patient's survival rate. Patients with low-level inflammation have a much better prognosis than those with high levels of inflammation.

Several articles in the medical journals over the years have consistently shown that people who use anti-inflammatory drugs such as Brufen, Ponstan and Nurofen for conditions such as osteoarthritis, rheumatic disorders or back pain have a much lower risk of developing cancer compared to people who do not take these drugs (Thun, 1996; Harris *et al.*, 1999; Nelson and Harris, 2000). Obviously, one cannot recommend such drugs to the general population as they have dangerous side effects: they all damage the lining of the gut and can cause intestinal bleeding. However, it supports the idea that anti-inflammatory is anti-cancer.

Research carried out at the University of California has carried on the good work begun in Scotland on the role that inflammation plays in cancer (Marx, 2004). In California, they have been able to isolate the single key inflammatory factor used by all cancers. It now appears that cancer cells rely heavily on a single factor called nuclear factor kappa B, or simply nuclear factor. In the scientific world it is now referred to as the black knight of cancer. It is the single most important chemical that promotes the growth and spread of cancer. Without nuclear factor, cancers would simply wither and die (Karin and Greten, 2005).

Table 3.2 is a summary of the types of cancer that have been identified as being associated with specific chronic inflammation.

Many of the preventive measures for cancer are really inhibitors of nuclear factor. Many anti-cancer foods, for example, act by blocking the action of this key molecule. Drug companies are presently spending millions of dollars looking for drugs that are capable of blocking nuclear factor. However, it is known in nutritional medicine that certain foods, such as those that contain omega 3 fatty acids and green tea, are well able to block this inflammatory factor.

Table 3.2: **Cancers Associated with Specific Chronic Inflammation**

Cancer	Chronic Inflammation
Oesophageal cancer	Barrett's oesophagus
Stomach cancer	Chronic gastritis
Colon cancer	Ulcerative colitis
Liver cancer	Chronic hepatitis
Bronchial cancer	Chronic bronchitis
Ovarian cancer	Pelvic inflammatory disease

SUMMARY

As I discussed in this chapter, not only do certain foods act as initiators of cancer but they also promote its growth and spread. However, certain foods, such as those containing omega 3, can also work to prevent cancer and its growth. So what we put into our bodies can be crucial when it comes to cancer. I will discuss the topic of food and diet in more detail in Chapter 5.

Pasteurised milk is a good example of a food that promotes the growth and spread of cancer. The solid scientific research supporting this idea has prompted Harvard Public Health Laboratory to remove dairy products from its food plate, which is used to promote a healthy diet.

Sugar, which stimulates the release not only of insulin but also of a substance called IGF (insulin-like growth factor), is known to promote the growth and spread of cancer. Many starchy food products, such as bread, pasta and pizza, do exactly the same thing. The advice to eat more starchy food is clearly wrong and is actually causing harm.

Another major factor that can promote the development of cancer is chronic inflammation. The level of inflammatory markers is now used worldwide as an indication of the aggression of a cancer and so is used to determine the prognosis. It has also been shown that anti-inflammatory measures, such as consuming foods containing omega 3, can prevent cancer from developing.

Chapter 4
The Importance of the Gut

There is no point in eating a very healthy diet if your gut is not functioning correctly. It's a bit like putting high-grade petrol into an engine that has a faulty carburettor. You will not get the desired result. So eating well and taking powerful nutritional supplements and top-of-the-range probiotics will not necessarily protect you against cancer. The most critical part of the body in terms of cancer prevention and general health is the gut.

When I was in medical school, my professor of medicine used to make the statement all the time that if you want to avoid ill health you should make sure your gut is working well. In other words, the key to good health is gut function. This makes absolute sense as the gut is the supply line for feeding the rest of body. If there's a problem with the supply line there will inevitably be a problem somewhere in the body as a consequence.

There are many things that can go wrong with your gut, from mouth ulcers at the top end to colitis at the bottom end. In this chapter I will deal with the more common disturbances in gut function. I will first address absorption issues as these are quite common.

ABSORPTION PROBLEMS

Leaky Gut Syndrome

This is a lot more common than you might imagine. It often occurs as a result of taking certain conventional drugs, especially painkillers or anti-inflammatories such as aspirin, Ponstan, Brufen and ibuprofen. These drugs all have the potential to damage the lining of the gut and cause inflammation of the gut wall.

Other drugs can also damage the gut lining, including antibiotics, especially broad spectrum antibiotics such as amoxycillin and tetracycline. The contraceptive pill, especially those with a high level of oestrogen, also has the potential to disturb gut function.

The digestive system is really a long tube like a hosepipe, the lining of which is only one cell thick. This makes the lining very vulnerable to damage. This lining blocks the entry of foreign substances into the bloodstream. When it is inflamed, the gut wall swells and this swelling allows the passage of stuff into the bloodstream that should not be there. In other words, the gut wall becomes leaky; hence the term 'leaky gut syndrome'.

A healthy gut lining allows only completely digested food to pass across into the bloodstream. The lining also functions as a barrier to prevent bacteria, foreign substances and partly digested food entering the bloodstream.

If these substances gain access to the bloodstream, your immune system will mount a reaction, a so-called allergic reaction. This is why leaky gut syndrome is associated with food allergies.

Apart from food allergies, leaky gut syndrome is associated with a range of medical problems, including serious disorders such as Crohn's disease and colitis. It is also associated with a range of disorders not often linked to the gut, such as asthma, as the following case history illustrates.

Case History – Belinda

Belinda was a very successful lawyer who worked for an international business consulting firm. She often had to travel across the world and seldom had time to rest. While on a visit to London, she developed a severe allergic-type reaction to something in her evening meal and had to be admitted to hospital with anaphylactic shock. All the medical tests done in London indicated a food allergy, which caused an asthma attack and shock, but they could not determine which food caused it. She was very scared afterwards as she knew she could go into a state of shock anywhere at any time.

I was suspicious that she had an underlying digestive problem and through a series of tests I discovered that she had severe leaky gut syndrome. Her gut was inflamed and was not preventing certain substances from crossing the gut wall. These substances, such as proteins or peptides (broken-down forms of protein), were entering her bloodstream instead of remaining in her gut to await digestion. Her body then reacted to the presence of these foreign substances by setting up an allergic reaction.

To treat Belinda, it was necessary for me to put her on a strict diet for a period of several months, which would allow her gut to heal. In addition, I put her on number of nutritional supplements, including glutamine, probiotics and digestive enzymes. I also recommended that she stop travelling as it would not be possible for her to follow the treatment regimen that I had proposed while keeping to her hectic schedule. Her boss agreed to base her at head office for one year to facilitate treatment. I also suggested that she go on a stress management course.

She has made excellent progress. She is now able to tolerate many of the foods she was allergic to, and, all in all, her level of health has improved remarkably. In addition, she has since left the corporate world and is now running a small farm.

In my clinical experience, the incidence of leaky gut syndrome is increasing and is also affecting younger age groups. The following case histories illustrate this.

Case History – John (six years old)

John had frequent bouts of diarrhoea for no apparent reason. All the conventional medical tests came back normal. I decided to do a gut permeability test, which revealed leaky gut syndrome. Treatment resolved the problem.

Case History – Ronan (sixteen years old)

Ronan also experienced bouts of diarrhoea with urgency; one bout occurred at school, causing him severe embarrassment. As a result, he was refusing to go to school, which is very understandable. Conventional drugs did not help. On testing him, I discovered that this young man had a leaky gut. Again, treatment resolved the issue.

Case History – Áine (20 years old)

Áine was experiencing bouts of diarrhoea with lots of mucus. A recent colonoscopy came back as normal, as did all her other tests. She also had leaky gut syndrome and again treatment resolved the problem.

Case History – James (29 years old)

James worked as an airline pilot and was suffering from excessive wind and bouts of loose motions. Tests revealed that he had leaky gut syndrome, and changes to his diet along with nutritional supplements resolved the problem.

The age of these patients ranged from six years old to late twenties. These patients hadn't lived long enough to have had much exposure to conventional drugs such as pain-killers and antibiotics; their medical histories also confirmed this. There has to be another gut irritant, an agent in our environment capable of causing significant inflammation of the small intestine of young people. Since this agent has a direct effect on the gut, it would have to be consumed. Some researchers in this area of medicine believe the culprit to be modern wheat, which contains a large amount of gluten.

All wheat contains gluten, which is actually a group of proteins. Rye and barley also contain gluten. However, in the Western world, wheat is the main source of gluten intake.

When I was a child growing up in Northern Ireland, wheat was a very tall plant. Most of the wheat grown today is only 30–60 centimetres tall, and as a consequence is called dwarf wheat. This dwarf wheat has been selected genetically because it produces much more food than the older type of wheat. In fact, it contains almost ten times more gluten than old wheat. It is gluten rich. This wheat is great for farmers as they get more money for their crops. It can feed more people, so this keeps the politicians and the UN Food and Agriculture Organization (FAO) happy. Its widespread use means that it's great for the *seed* producers, and because it requires more spraying of pesticides it means greater profits for the chemical companies.

Everyone is excited about modern wheat as it *seems* to have been a major advance in food production. So much was thought of this advance that Norman Borlaug, the American scientist who developed dwarf wheat, won a Nobel Prize for his efforts as well as a Congressional Gold Medal. The problem was that no one thought of testing this significantly altered wheat on humans. The assumption was that it was sufficiently like old wheat so as not to lead to any major health risks.

This assumption appears to be wrong. It *seems* that there is a much greater sensitivity to wheat among the general population compared to thirty years ago. For example, coeliac disease, which is a condition in which you react to gluten, is an inherited condition and so the incidence should remain pretty constant over time. Instead, it has quadrupled in my lifetime and is continuing to rise. This clearly indicates that there is an environmental factor at work.

On a personal note, I have never *seen* so much sensitivity to gluten in my thirty years of treating gut problems as I do now. Nor have I *seen* as many young people being affected, as the above case histories illustrate. If modern wheat has up to ten times more gluten in it than old wheat and if your gut is in any way sensitive to gluten, you will most definitely react.

One of the consequences of coeliac disease is malnourishment as a result of impaired absorption of nutrients across the gut wall. This puts the body at risk of infection and a range of other problems. If you do not absorb sufficient levels of antioxidants, you have diminished protection, not just against viruses and bacteria but also against carcinogenic chemicals. In other words, you are more at risk of cancer.

This also applies to anyone with gut absorption problems. Leaky gut syndrome should therefore be taken seriously, very seriously. It has huge consequences for the rest of your body, especially your immunity. If you don't look after your gut, your body will not function correctly. You may be eating the healthiest diet on planet Earth but you will not get the benefits if you have an absorption problem.

Leaky gut syndrome is now so prevalent in the Western world, affecting younger and younger age groups, that I test almost everyone who comes to *see* me. The test is very easy to perform and can be done at home with the correct kit. It involves swallowing a watery substance containing eleven different-sized molecules, and then collecting all the urine that you pass over a six-hour period. If too many of the molecules appear in the urine this suggests leaky gut syndrome – because it shows that the wall of your gut has become inflamed, so allowing things into the bloodstream that can be harmful. If too few of the molecules appear in the urine, you may be suffering from malabsorption, which I discuss below.

For example, Figure 4.1 shows how protein in food is broken down by the digestive tract. First, it is chopped into smaller bits, called peptides, in the stomach. These peptides then pass into the small intestine and are broken down into even smaller bits, called amino acids, which are then absorbed into the body and reassembled to make proteins that the body needs.

Figure 4.1: Protein Digestion

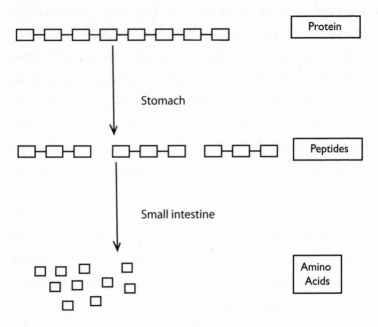

Protein: A long chain of amino acids.
Peptide: A short chain of amino acids.

If you have a leaky gut, peptides can leak across the gut wall. However, these peptides are useless to the body. Therefore, you will not get the benefit of the protein you have just consumed. In addition, the immune system will react to these peptides and cause an allergic reaction. If this happens every day, your immune system will become depleted.

So, a leaky gut is not some minor gut condition that causes bloating, flatulence and so on after a meal. It is not a condition that is self-limiting and will eventually heal on its own. It requires diagnosis and treatment until fully healed. Treatment involves dietary changes as well as taking nutritional supplements.

Malabsorption

Malabsorption is as serious a condition as leaky gut syndrome, if not more so. Malabsorption means that a reduced amount of nutrients are able to cross the gut wall. It results in malnutrition, initially affecting the visible or external tissues of the body: the hair, skin and nails. Hair becomes brittle and dry, and nails become weak and brittle, and can develop white spots and ridging. The skin at the base of the fingernails can become swollen and inflamed and can break down.

It's generally thought that white spots on your fingernails are caused by a lack of calcium. However, these white spots actually indicate a deficiency in either zinc or selenium. This deficiency can be due to a gut absorption problem such as malabsorption but can also be due to a zinc deficiency in the soil in the area where you live or where the food you buy is from.

Excluding problems due to zinc deficiency in the soil, the most common reason for white spots on your fingernails is zinc deficiency associated with an absorption problem in the gut. Zinc is important for your immune system, and so a deficiency can weaken your immunity and make you more vulnerable, not only to infection but to cancer as well.

Of the common gut disorders that may result in malabsorption, the two most frequently encountered are coeliac disease and Crohn's disease. Both of these diseases lead to damage to the wall of the gut and, in so doing, reduce the surface area available for absorption of nutrients.

Coeliac disease is particularly common among the Celtic race, including the Scots, the Irish, the Welsh and the Bretons. The Celts have the highest incidence of coeliac disease in the world and the greatest sensitivity to gluten. We do not tolerate wheat very well, especially modern wheat as I explained in the previous section.

The geneticists have had a field day playing around with the genes found in wheat. They have altered its genetic composition so much that the plant is unrecognisable. It looks completely different and is completely different. It has been altered so much that the head of the plant produces nearly ten times more starch and ten times more gluten than that of old wheat. There is no doubt that modern wheat is a major agricultural/genetic achievement. It has indeed fed more people worldwide. The only problem with modern wheat (apart from polluting the environment with chemicals) is that the geneticists forgot to try it out on people to *see* if it caused any problems.

Other gut-related disorders that may lead to malabsorption include pancreatitis, which can reduce the number of digestive enzymes available to digest food properly. Undigested or partly digested protein will putrefy in the gut in the same way that meat decays. Putrefied protein is very toxic to the body and will set up an inflammatory condition in the gut wall.

Other causes of malabsorption include the presence of parasites such as *Giardia lamblia*, or heavy worm infestations that take a share of your food. Significant disturbances in the gut flora may also cause malabsorption, which is why I recommend a suitable probiotic to virtually all my patients. I discuss probiotics and their function in more detail in my book *Antibiotics: Are They Curing Us or Killing Us?* (2014).

There are also a host of non-gut-related conditions that can result in malabsorption, such as thyroid abnormalities (hyperthyroidism and hypothyroidism), lactose intolerance, soya milk intolerance and fructose intolerance.

Like leaky gut syndrome, malabsorption must be taken very seriously as it impairs the transport of important nutrients across the gut wall, thus weakening the immune system. Again, the treatment of malabsorption involves dietary changes (*see* Chapter 6) and the use of a number of nutritional supplements. You should repeat the gut permeability test outlined in the section on leaky gut syndrome above to ensure progress.

Gut Fermentation

Fermentation is a natural process that occurs if you mix carbohydrate with yeast at around 37 degrees Celsius, or body temperature. The carbohydrate can be in the form of sugar, such as table sugar or glucose, or it can be in the form of starch, such as bread, porridge, pasta, potatoes or rice. The key elements in making wine or cider or beer are a form of carbohydrate, sufficient levels of yeast and the right temperature.

It should be no big surprise, then, to learn that fermentation can occur in your digestive tract as well as in a distillery. Two of the three key requisites are present in most people – intake of carbohydrate and body temperature. While few people have sufficient levels of yeast in their digestive tract for fermentation to occur. People who have taken many courses of antibiotics, are under chronic stress or have a significant disturbance in the bacterial flora can go on to develop gut fermentation.

Gut fermentation means that the sugar or starch you eat is converted to alcohol. It is clearly a malfunction of the gut and puts the body under great stress. It tends to occur in the small intestine. Impairment of the function of the small intestine is far more serious than impairment of the large intestine, as the small intestine is responsible for the digestion and absorption of food, both of which are critical to your overall health. It is the critical supply line of nutrients to your body to keep your organs ticking. You cannot survive without the small intestine; by contrast, people can and do survive and thrive without a large intestine, should they need it removed surgically in such conditions as ulcerative colitis or bowel cancer.

Impairment of the small intestine is a slow, insidious process and can go unnoticed for a long time. Unlike the skin, which is well supplied with nerves and warns you very quickly when damage occurs, the small intestine is poorly supplied with nerves and is therefore less able to warn you when things go wrong.

Symptoms of Fermentation

Some of the symptoms of fermentation are obvious. If the energy-giving foods are being hijacked and converted to alcohol, you will suffer not only from a lack of energy but you may have a drunk or hungover feeling. Having said that, the symptoms can be few or many, very subtle or apparent; they can be related to the digestive tract or to other parts of the body. Let's look at the digestive symptoms first.

Anyone who has made homemade wine or beer will tell you that the top can blow off the bottle or container they are using. This is caused by a gas that is produced as a byproduct of fermentation. The gas is carbon dioxide. When carbon dioxide is produced in the gut in large quantities, it will be released from the gut at the upper end as burping or belching and at the lower end as flatulence.

That's not to say that all cases of excessive wind in the gut are the result of fermentation, as there are many other reasons for excessive flatulence. It is merely one of a complex of symptoms associated with this maldigestion of carbohydrate.

Here are a few case histories to illustrate other parts of the symptom complex.

Case History – Kevin: Bad Breath

Kevin was twenty-five years old and was suffering from bad breath or halitosis.

His family and girlfriend had told him to get help for it; hence his visit to me. He was a relaxed kind of guy but was under a lot of stress as he was trying to work and study at the same time and therefore had little relaxation time in his day. He was a full-time student at university and also had a part-time job as a waiter in a busy restaurant. Because of his hectic schedule he had an erratic eating pattern, snatching meals where he could. Much of what he ate consisted of starch: bread, pasta, potatoes, hamburgers and hot dogs. He ate very little fresh food.

Kevin also complained of having a strong body odour on occasion as well as very heavy sweating, especially at night. He often had to change his pajamas in the middle of the night. His hands and feet could also sometimes be cold and clammy.

On examining him, I found he had a thick white coating on his tongue, his hands and feet were indeed cold and clammy, and his abdomen was very tender, especially the area around the belly button where the small intestine sits. He also had a nasty case of athlete's foot, which is a fungal infection of the skin between the toes and on the sole of the foot.

I did a number of tests on Kevin and these revealed a significant yeast overgrowth in his gut as well as gut fermentation. Further medical history from Kevin revealed that he had been put on antibiotics for over two years in his late teens because he suffered from acne. This explained why he had such a disturbance to the bacterial population (see Chapter 2 of my book Hard to Stomach*).*

Treatment involved avoiding all sugars and starch, and taking an anti-fungal supplement as well as a good probiotic. Gradually all of Kevin's symptoms started to resolve, although it took four months for him to fully recover.

Kevin's case history is very interesting in that he did not present with classic gut symptoms such as wind, bloating, heartburn and so on. Rather, he was complaining of bad breath, body odour and heavy sweating at night. So just because there is an absence of gut symptoms, it does not mean all is well in the gut. This is a mistake that many patients make, and many doctors do too. Remember, the gut is poorly supplied with nerves and so is less able to wave a warning flag. Many times I have encountered patients who tell me their gut is fine, but when I examine them and do tests, it clearly is not fine. This is why you really need to have gut function tests, as described above and in detail in my book *Hard to Stomach*, done every couple of years if you are serious about preventing cancer. Testing is critical for unearthing problems such as fermentation, dysbiosis (disturbance in the gut flora), putre-faction and absorption problems, as all these can weaken the body and add to its toxicity level, so predisposing it to cancer.

Sometimes patients with a gut fermentation problem do have stomach symptoms, as the next two case histories illustrate. These symptoms include excessive wind, trapped wind, bloating, gurgling sounds, cramps and nausea, especially upon waking.

Case History – Barry: Belching

Barry, who was forty-two, came to see me complaining of excessive belching. He said that he was belching up to eighty times a day and that it was noticeably worse after eating. He found it very embarrassing as he had to deal with business clients every day and some of them had commented on his habit of belching. He had a very stressful job dealing with financial investments on the internet, and because he had become self-employed in the past two years, he had to work very long hours and often at weekends as well. He had been to his family doctor, who had done various tests on him, all of which came back fine. The doctor told him to take a holiday, which he said would solve the problem.

Because I have had many years of dealing with similar cases to Barry's, it was quite easy to diagnose what was wrong within a few minutes of speaking to him. Unfortunately, not all patients are as easy to diagnose as Barry. On examining him, I discovered that his abdomen was distended, and when I tapped it with my fingers it was very resonant. His stomach was excessively noisy as well.

I asked him to do a test for me to confirm the diagnosis. Two days later, the results came back confirming that he did indeed have gut fermentation. I then treated him over the coming months with a fermentation control diet and various supplements. After the first month of treatment, he showed remarkable improvement, and from then onwards the belching only recurred when he broke his diet. He began to notice the very detrimental effects of sugar in particular.

In addition to reduced belching, he also noticed that he had increased energy and he was sleeping much better. He was waking in the mornings feeling refreshed and not hungover as before. After four months I repeated the test and showed him the results, which showed a significant improvement. When he saw the improved results, he was very happy and was motivated to continue treatment. A few months later, he was stronger still and feeling full of energy. He told me he hadn't felt as well in years. He then decided to hire an assistant to allow him more time with his family. Another repeat test indicated that he was no longer fermenting food and so he could then resume a normal diet.

The next case history also relates to a gut symptom – excessive bowel sounds or gurgling sounds.

Case History – Gary: Gurgling Sounds

Gary was thirty-four years old and married with three children. His wife complained that his tummy was always making noises, which was most noticeable in bed at night. She also told him that his body was extremely warm, describing him as an electric radiator and saying that it was uncomfortable to lie close to him. For a long time, she had been telling Gary to go to see a doctor about these symptoms, but he did not consider them to be serious enough. More recently, he began to get boils that were quite big and painful, and some of them developed into abscesses that had to be drained in hospital.

Gary was convinced that there was nothing wrong with his

digestive system, and when I suggested a possible link between his noisy tummy and his skin problems he laughed and dismissed the idea as ludicrous. I told him that I would bet that I was right and if his test results came back normal I would refer him to another doctor. He agreed to give it a try as he had nothing to lose.

When I examined him, I found that his ribcage angle was approximately 120 degrees instead of 30 degrees and he had obvious ribcage humping. His abdomen was acutely tender on palpation, and while listening with the stethoscope I can honestly say I have never heard a noisier digestive tract.

Gary lost the bet as his test results indicated a marked fermentation problem. He still did not believe that this had anything to do with his boils and abscesses but was willing to give the treatment a trial for one month. His wife was very supportive and made sure that he ate only what he was allowed. She also made sure that he took all of the supplements as prescribed.

One month later he was amazed at the improvements – the gurgling had stopped, his bowel habit had improved, his wife reported that his body temperature was more normal and he did not have one new boil. He was so impressed that he started referring other people to me.

What is most interesting about Gary's case is the fact that his body was producing so much heat. When fermentation is well advanced, a lot of heat can be produced, which can be very uncomfortable. Gary told me that he preferred to sleep with only one sheet at night, even when the bedroom temperature was low, and that he insisted on keeping the window open at night despite his wife complaining of the cold. Heat is a byproduct of fermentation. Anyone who has made homemade wine will also tell you that the bottle or container can get warm. As the yeast converts the starch or sugar to alcohol, carbon dioxide gas is released and heat is produced.

Gut fermentation is a bit like having your own personal brewery – no need to go to the local pub when your body is supplying you with alcohol after you consume carbohydrate foods. When your body is exposed to alcohol over a period of time, certain additional symptoms can occur. Since alcohol is a diuretic, you may find yourself passing water more frequently and you may wake at night to urinate. In addition, you may wake in the morning feeling groggy and tired, and maybe with a headache. This hungover feeling is a cardinal symptom of gut fermentation. Often a patient will report that it can take up to an hour for these hungover symptoms to decrease. The next case history is an example of precisely this.

Case History – Sinead: Exhaustion upon Waking

Sinead was eighteen years old when she came to see me complaining of low energy. She told me that she was waking up most mornings feeling drugged and that it took her about an hour to come alive. Her energy would dip in the afternoon and she often had to go to bed early in the evening as she felt tired. Because this energy pattern is very uncommon among teenagers, who tend to have high natural energy, I proceeded to ask about other symptoms so that I could make a tentative diagnosis.

After questioning her and examining her, I was still unsure as to the root cause of her energy problem. Tests revealed that she had low iron stores, marginally low thyroid function and gut fermentation. I treated the fermentation problem and gave her a non-constipating iron supplement. Within one month of starting treatment, her energy was back to normal. I advised her to stay on treatment and, in the long term, not to eat her main meal in the evening, as she had been doing, and also to avoid all starch – rice, pasta, potatoes, bread – in the evening.

Sinead continued with treatment and showed further improvement. Three months later, repeat tests were normal and so we were able to stop treatment. She could now maintain good energy levels throughout the day and was waking each morning feeling refreshed and alert.

Low energy can have more than one cause in the same patient, so it is important to look for multiple causes. These include vitamin and mineral deficiencies – especially of vitamin B12 and iron – low thyroid function, dysbiosis and gut fermentation.

If a person with a digestive disturbance consumes sugar or starch – starch is a long chain of glucose molecules – the glucose may ferment to form alcohol, which as we know is gut fermentation. This alcohol is then absorbed across the gut wall and intoxicates the person – this is called auto-intoxication. In other words, toxic chemicals are being produced *inside* the body as distinct from chemicals entering the body from outside. So the symptom of feeling hungover or drugged upon waking is strongly suggestive of gut fermentation.

Alcohol by auto-intoxication has pretty much the same effects on your body as going to the pub on a regular basis. Chronic alcohol exposure generates the production of fat in the body. This fat gets deposited in various parts of the body and causes problems. It can be deposited in the liver, causing inflammation (hepatitis) and ultimately cirrhosis, and later still cancer. Fat deposited around the abdomen results in the classic beer belly. This fat that is deposited in various organs and around the abdomen generates the production of oestrogen. This hormone can then promote the growth of oestrogen-dependent cancers such as breast cancer.

So you *see* that correcting a digestive disturbance such as fermentation is important if you wish to avoid cancer. All patients who have cancer or have had it in the past must be checked for gut problems, as these are a less obvious cause of exposure to toxic chemicals.

Putrefaction

The maldigestion of protein can lead to putrefaction. If you leave a piece of meat sitting on your kitchen table for a certain amount of time, it will begin to putrefy or decay. This renders the meat very toxic, which can upset the gut significantly, as you may have experienced after eating some dodgy food in a restaurant.

Putrefaction of protein results in the generation of nasty chemicals such as indican, putrescine, nervine and cadaverine. The presence of these chemicals can be tested for by means of an early morning specimen of urine.

Putrefactive chemicals such as indican and putrescine can irritate and inflame the gut, causing symptoms such as nausea, heartburn, indigestion, constipation or diarrhoea. These chemicals are quite nasty and if the condition is left untreated, they may end up causing bowel cancer (cancer of the colon).

The presence of these chemicals in your system would suggest that you are not digesting protein correctly and so you should reduce or avoid animal protein and take digestive enzymes. There are basically two types of digestive enzyme supplements. The first one contains betaine hydrochloride, which supplements stomach acid, and the second type does not contain betaine hydrochloride. The former type is for people with low stomach acid, whereas the second type is for patients with normal or high levels of stomach acid.

Putrefaction can cause cancer by favouring the overgrowth of bad bacteria in the gut, such as *Bacteroides spp.* These bacteria are able to convert bile salts into very toxic substances, which then promote the growth of cancer. *Bacteroids spp* can also break down the vitamins you consume in food, rendering you deficient in these vitamins. If these bacteria break down vitamin B12, you may suffer from symptoms such as fatigue (low physical energy), depression (low mental energy), and tingling in the hands and feet.

Therefore, if you consume a lot of animal protein and/or have a low level of stomach acid (your GP can tell you if this is the case), and you suffer from abdominal symptoms, it may be wise to get checked out if you are serious about preventing cancer. Toxicity can be lurking in your gut and can go unnoticed for a long time.

DYSBIOSIS AND BOWEL CANCER

Digestive problems are much more common than you may realise and can affect any age group. I spent most of my working life in different parts of Africa where digestive problems are rare and are usually caused by parasites and worms. In the Western world, because of the use of conventional drugs, especially antibiotics, and also because living in our society can be stress-inducing, gut problems are infinitely more common.

Never underestimate the damage that gut problems can do to your general health. Not only can they deplete your energy and vitality, but they can also end up causing cancer. Years ago when I was studying medicine, I remember being taught about the connection between bowel cancer and disturbances in the bacterial population of the digestive system. Let's explore this concept a little further now.

Case History – John: Colitis

John was a research scientist in the pharmaceutical industry and found his job incredibly stressful. He was happily married with two young children and loved his family very much. He had read my book Hard to Stomach and he came to see me in the hope that I could help him reverse his colitis.

John was thirty-three years old and had been having ongoing health issues since his early twenties. These issues were mainly gut-related in that he had acute bouts of severe bloating, wind and pain. These bouts became more frequent over the years and more recently they were associated with diarrhoea, which occasionally had blood and mucus in it.

His family doctor had referred him to a gastroenterologist who did various tests and concluded that he had mild colitis (inflammation of the colon or large bowel). Both doctors explained that this condition put him at a higher risk of developing bowel cancer. This scared John as he had a young family, and it made him determined to leave no stone unturned in an attempt to reverse his condition.

He wanted me to do gut function tests for him so that he could see what was underlying the colitis symptoms. I agreed *to do a range of tests for him and these revealed very marked dysbiosis. He had been on tetracycline (a broad-spectrum antibiotic) for the best part of three years in his early twenties as he suffered from acne. He had a recurrence of the acne a few years later and was prescribed tetracycline once again. This was most likely the cause of the severe dysbiosis.*

I put him on treatment immediately and within days he began to improve. First, his stool became more solid and better formed and the bleeding stopped. Then his gut became much calmer with less bloating and wind. What was more noticeable to him was his mood and energy levels, both of which improved. His skin became clearer as well. Six months later, a repeat test confirmed an improvement. However, I advised him to stay on probiotics long term to ensure that the bacterial flora remained normal.

One year later, he had a repeat colonoscopy performed by the same gastroenterologist, who declared that there was now no evidence of colitis. He was elated with the progress he had made, but despite this he has stuck rigidly to his diet and takes a probiotic and flaxseed every day. He is really committed to staying healthy and well.

It is a gross understatement to say that the bacterial population of the body is important. This population forms 90 per cent of your body; the other 10 per cent is formed of human cells. Safe to say then that each of us is composed mainly of bacteria – a strange thought! Just because we cannot *see* these bacteria with the naked eye doesn't make them any less real.

This coating of bacterial cells covers the skin and lines the tubes of the body: the digestive tract and airway, as well as the vagina in females. It forms the first line of defence against microbes and toxins, and as such forms an integral part of the immune system (*see* Chapter 6 for more about bacteria and their benefits).

We can replace the good bacteria every day, with soured milk, buttermilk or live yoghurt. When raw milk is left to stand or used to make yoghurt, the living bacteria in the milk (lactic acid bacteria or lactobacilli) multiply and curd the milk. This is why buttermilk, soured milk products and live yoghurt form such a critical element of one's diet. Pasteurised milk, on the other hand, does not have living bacteria in it and so is useless at replacing the good bacteria.

Therefore, if you wish to replace the bacterial population daily, do not rely on commercial yoghurts found in supermarkets. The majority of them are made with pasteurised milk. Don't be fooled by statements such as 'Made with live cultures' or 'Made with organic milk'. The yoghurt may have had live cultures or been from an organic source, but once it was heat treated, all the bacteria would have died.

Because of the association between consumption of pasteurised dairy products and cancer (*see* Chapter 3), it is wise to either avoid dairy completely or to use only raw milk fresh from the cow. However, if using raw milk, check that the cattle producing the milk have been checked for tuberculosis and brucellosis.

The main benefit of consuming live yoghurt or soured milk is that they contain bacteria that produce acids, such as lactic acid, which inhibit the growth of bad bacteria. Good bacteria in live yoghurt or soured milk also play a critical role in the digestion of food and in the elimination of waste from the bowel. A disturbance in the bacterial flora will often result in constipation or diarrhoea, and if left untreated may end up causing bowel cancer.

Probably the most important function of the bacterial flora is to interact with the white blood cells. Researchers in Japan found that supplementation with beneficial bacteria increased the lymphocyte (white blood cell) count and in particular increased the number of killer T cells (Sugawara *et al.*, 2006). In other words, the bacterial flora are in constant communication with your white blood cells to alert them to danger and prime them for action.

The place to begin cancer prevention is with the bacterial population of your body. If it is disturbed, as *seen* in test results as either dysbiosis or gut fermentation, or you have putrefaction, then treat these conditions and use a daily probiotic either in capsule form or as live yoghurt. This will not only assist with better digestion but will help to ensure a healthy immune system able to deal with environmental toxins and act as a powerful defence against cancer.

SUMMARY

Disturbances in the gut have major detrimental effects on all aspects of human health. There is an epidemic of digestive problems in the modern world. Put another way, almost any complaint that a patient presents with to a medical professional should be treated as a symptom of a digestive problem until proven otherwise. That's how common digestive problems are and how often they can display non-digestive symptoms. I now routinely do digestive tests on all my patients almost irrespective of their complaint.

I begin by taking a detailed medical history, including asking about emotional health. Then I do a thorough examination followed by gut function tests and toxicity tests, and I test for particular vitamin/mineral levels where appropriate. In this way, I get a complete picture of the person's medical condition and how best I can assist. I do this for both children and adults. I try to make the tests as non-invasive as possible and as simple as possible, and in the case of children I avoid referring them for blood tests unless absolutely necessary.

Some of the most common conditions that these tests show are disturbances in the bacterial flora (dysbiosis), gut fermentation and leaky gut syndrome. Other gut problems such as malabsorption and putrefaction are less common. The presence of toxic metals, some of which are carcinogenic, is not uncommon. Vitamin and mineral deficiencies, especially among children, are alarmingly frequent.

The prevention of cancer begins with the gut and most especially with the bacterial flora. I would again urge you to have gut function and toxicity tests done regularly, like having routine blood tests done. That way you can keep your gut healthy and will be less likely to discover a tumour further down the line.

Chapter 5
Diet

Your diet is now regarded by many as the most important determinant in whether you will develop cancer. What we eat and drink enters our bodies and interacts with our epigenomes (receptors on the DNA and its protein framework – *see* Chapter 1); therefore what we consume has the power to switch on certain genes and dampen or switch off other genes. A healthy diet therefore plays a pivotal role in the prevention of cancer.

In discussing diet, I will look at the foods we should reduce or avoid and explain the scientific reason why. Later in the chapter, I will look at the foods we should include in our diet and explain how these foods act as anti-cancer agents. But first I would like to tell an unusual story about a very interesting Canadian scientist.

Professor Richard Béliveau is currently the director of the Molecular Medicine Laboratory and a researcher in the Department of Neurosurgery at Notre-Dame Hospital, Quebec. In the early 1980s, he was a professor of biochemistry at the University of Montreal and his main area of interest was analysing how anti-cancer medicines work at a biochemical level. He worked with many of the major drug companies in the world, trying to give these companies insights into how best to develop new anti-cancer drugs. He worked within the grounds of the university and so never met a person who actually had cancer in the course of his research.

Then all of that changed. His laboratory was relocated to the children's hospital in Montreal, which was also part of the university. His neighbour in these new premises was the professor in charge of blood cancers such as leukaemia. In one of the first conversations between the two men, this professor asked Richard if he could find a way of reducing the toxicity of conventional anti-cancer drugs. The professor was an open-minded man and he asked Richard to come up with something, anything that would help the children.

Every day Richard had to walk through the department where these children were being treated and every day he was asked by the parents of these children for help. The most difficult thing for him was interacting with the children themselves. This daily exposure to the human reality of cancer had a profound effect on Richard and drove him to find answers. Unlike the doctors treating these children, Richard had the time and scientific knowledge to discover innovative treatments.

He set about trawling through the vast amount of scientific data on cancer and came upon a very interesting article in the well-respected journal *Nature*. The article had been written by two researchers at the world-famous Karolinska Institute, Sweden and described how green tea was able to block the development of new blood vessels necessary for the growth of cancer (Cao and Cao, 1999). It drew on the premise that places where green tea was drunk frequently had significantly lower instances of cancer. This was confirmed by other data Richard uncovered. He could not believe that such a simple dietary change could have such a profound effect, yet all the data supported it. It *see*med too simple to be true (Béliveau and Gingas, 2006).

This was both an interesting and a hopeful discovery, but following such a line of research could also prove challenging. The fact that conventional medicine and the pharmaceutical companies, with whom Richard had such a close working relationship, did not accept nutrition as important in cancer therapy threatened his professional career. Despite this, the human need that he witnessed every day in the hospital convinced him to follow the path of nutrition and learn more.

He then began to wonder if other foods also had such remarkable anti-cancer properties. If so, they could offer a non-toxic alternative to drugs for the children he saw every day. His laboratory of molecular medicine, with over fifty full-time researchers, was now about to take a big risk. They were going to devote some of their time, energy and money to a project that would not generate income – food items cannot be patented and so no profit would be generated.

Over the following weeks and months, Professor Béliveau developed a list of foods that could protect the body against cancer. This research went hand in hand with an under-standing of what foods could have a negative effect on the body and play a role in the development of cancer. He quickly began to *see* the harm being done by common foods in a Western diet. He therefore thought that the advice he would give to the parents of the sick children should begin with what foods to exclude from their diet. That is where I will begin as well.

FOODS TO ELIMINATE FROM THE DIET

The original diet of humankind was similar to that of very isolated peoples today, such as the Sami people of Northern Europe or the Inuit of northern Canada. The diet of these people includes reindeer meat, reindeer milk, fish and some fruit and berries, but little in the way of vegetables, as it is too cold up close to the Arctic to grow vegetables, and definitely no cereals and no sugar. Tribal cultures further south on the planet, such as the Fulani of West Africa or the Maasai of East Africa, also have a very basic diet but with a bit more variety, including vegetables and a wider range of fruit. However, as these people are nomadic, they do not stay in one place for long enough to grow crops, especially cereals such as corn, rice or wheat.

Similarly, the primitive diet was based mostly on animal produce – animal fat and protein – and occasional fruits. So it was a very simple, basic diet, and was based on a nomadic existence. It is no surprise then that our genome or genetic material has adapted to digest these very natural foods. They are the foods that cause people the least difficulty.

About 10,000 years ago, humans settled and began to grow crops such as wheat. More recently, due to the exporting opportunities opened up by sea travel and due to the necessities of warfare, tinned foods and other forms of processed food were developed. These processed foods are often produced with high levels of sugar.

High Glycaemic Index Foods: Sugar and Wheat

In Chapter 3, I identified sugar and wheat as being high-GI foods. Now I would like to discuss in more detail their connection with cancer.

Sugar

Sugar is everywhere in Western foodstuffs. In fact, it can be found in virtually every processed food in your local super-market. This signifies a massive change in the human diet in recent times, in fact the biggest change in human history.

As outlined in Chapters 1 and 3, the first important principle to understand is that cancer feeds on sugar. If you do not feed it sugar, it cannot grow. We are now beginning to understand the effects that sugar has on the body and how it affects the development and growth of cancer.

Back in 1924 German scientist Professor Otto Heinrich Warburg first showed that the growth of malignant tumours is largely dependent on glucose. He showed that healthy cells need oxygen as well as glucose to release energy. He also showed that cancer cells function very differently from normal cells in that they do not require oxygen and only require glucose to release energy.

Professor Warburg went on to show that cancer cells could release energy from glucose anywhere in the cell, whereas normal cells release energy in the mitochondria only. Therefore, he was the first to show that cancer cells operate in a very different way to normal cells (Warburg, 1956).

As outlined in Chapter 3, if we eat foods containing sugar or starch (wheat, rice, porridge, potatoes), which is composed of glucose, the level of glucose rises in our bloodstream. As a result, many carbohydrate foods – sugars and starches – are said to have a high GI. Because too much glucose in the bloodstream is quite dangerous, the body releases insulin, which pushes glucose out of the bloodstream and into the cells. At the same time that insulin is released another molecule called insulin-like growth factor (IGF) is also released, which stimulates the cells to grow and divide. So, glucose ends up feeding cells and making them grow faster.

This has been borne out by science. Today we know that secretion of both insulin and IGF directly stimulates the growth of cancer cells, as reported in the *Journal of Cancer Research and Clinical Oncology* (Grothey *et al.*, 1999). We also know that insulin and IGF can enhance the ability of cancer cells to invade surrounding normal tissue, that is, to spread locally. This has been reported in the journal *Cancer Research* (Long *et al.*, 1998).

IGF doesn't only promote the growth and spread of cancer. Scientific research has shown that it reduces the effectiveness of chemotherapy. When researchers injected breast cancer cells into laboratory mice, they found that these cancer cells were less responsive to various anti-cancer drugs (chemotherapy) in mice whose diet was rich in sugar. So a diet high in sugar can also make cancer cells less susceptible to chemotherapy. Therefore, not only does diet play a role in the growth of cancer but it also affects the treatment of it (Dunn *et al.*, 1997). This discovery has led to drug companies conducting research into drugs that block the release of IGF. But wouldn't it be easier to just reduce our intake of foods with a high GI and replace them with low-glycaemic foods?

Now you can understand why practitioners of natural medicine are so against anything in the diet that raises blood glucose levels. They all advocate a low-GI diet containing foods that have little or no effect on insulin and IGF.

I personally do not abstain from sugar completely but I do keep its intake to a minimum – once a week, a piece of apple pie or a slice of Bakewell tart goes down a treat. We are all human and if there is a big juicy cake put in front of us, most of us will fall victim to the temptation. It is entirely up to you how you live your life, as long as you are informed.

However, having said that, remember that sugar is highly addictive. In my book *Good Food* I described how I became addicted to sugar as a youngster while working in my neighbour's grocery shop during the school holidays. I was paid in chocolate bars and fruit gums instead of money. I quickly became addicted and used to suffer episodes of hypoglycemia. If I had known then what I know now about sugar, I would have opted for cash.

All the scientific data collected to date points to sugar as the main culprit in the diet, yet it is the most ubiquitous molecule in the Western diet. When Asians, such as Indians or Chinese, follow their traditional low-sugar diet they have up to ten times fewer hormonally driven cancers – breast, prostate, endometrial and testicular – compared to Asians who adopt a Western high-sugar diet. The higher your insulin and IGF levels, the higher the risk of developing cancer.

In the 1980s and 1990s, artificial sweeteners became widely available and may well explain the increase in blood cancers since then, in particular leukaemia, lymphoma and myeloma (Schernhammer *et al.*, 2012). I have discussed these sweeteners in detail in my book *Good Food*. My advice is to avoid all artificial sweeteners – aspartame (Nutrasweet or Equal), sucralose (Splenda) and acesulfame K.

Wheat
Let's deal with the essential difference between refined flour and unrefined flour before we discuss the cancer risks of consuming wheat.

White bread is mostly made from refined wheat flour. Unrefined whole-wheat flour contains a lot of good stuff such as protein, starch, fibre, vitamins and minerals, as well as enzymes that help you digest it. Refined white flour has only the protein and starch, which have been chemically treated. To digest refined flour, your body has to supply its own vitamins and minerals and enzymes. In other words, refined flour puts demands on your body and if you do not have sufficient levels of vitamins or minerals you will have great difficulty digesting it. For example, B vitamins are essential for the metabolism of wheat but these B vitamins are removed in the refining process. Thus, if your body doesn't have enough B vitamins, you won't be able to metabolise the wheat and get energy from it. Refined flour places a big burden on your body. It ends up being poorly digested and setting up an inflammatory reaction in the gut.

Apart from being a high-GI food, and hence a stimulator of IGF, wheat can also cause chronic inflammation. As discussed in Chapter 4, chronic inflammation anywhere in the body has the potential to turn cancerous. If you have a long-standing gut problem associated with wheat consumption then you are at a higher risk of developing cancer somewhere along the digestive tract. For example, those who suffer from coeliac disease and do not follow a strict gluten-free diet are more likely to develop cancer.

Studies comparing the incidence of cancer in coeliacs compared to non-coeliacs showed that those in the coeliac group were 30 per cent more likely to develop some form of cancer. In addition, one in every thirty-three coeliacs developed cancer within the three-year period of observation. Most of the cancers were located in the gut (West *et al.*, 2004).

This amazing research has been confirmed by a study carried out among 12,000 coeliacs in Sweden, which also showed a 30 per cent greater likelihood of coeliacs develop-ing cancer than non-coeliacs. However, what is interesting is that this increased risk is totally reversible if the coeliac abstains from gluten (wheat, rye and barley) and follows a strict gluten- free diet (Askling, 2002).

If coeliac disease as well as gluten intolerance – a condition whereby you can't tolerate gluten but do not have coeliac disease – is not diagnosed and therefore not treated, you run the risk of developing non-Hodgkin's lymphoma of the small intestine. This cancer is particularly common among coeliacs. However, the risk reduces once you avoid gluten, especially wheat. Other common cancers that affect coeliacs include cancer of the throat, mouth and oesophagus, as well as cancer of the large intestine, pancreas and liver.

What's staggering is that most coeliacs and most people with gluten intolerance go undiagnosed – depending on which book you read, this figure could be up to 90 per cent. As I mentioned, the Irish and other Celts have the highest incidence of these conditions on the planet. Undiagnosed inflammation of the gut can lead to cancer. If you wish to avoid cancer, get yourself checked for any digestive issues.

Bread made with white refined flour is popularly considered to be a high-GI food, while whole-wheat bread is counted among the low-GI foods. This is not accurate. A study carried out by the University of Toronto in 1981 listed the GI of whole-wheat bread as 72 and that of white bread as 69 (Jenkins *et al.*, 1981). As you can *see*, both are very high and so both should be listed as high-GI foods.

Table 5.1 contains a list of high-GI and low-GI foods. I would suggest avoiding all of the foods in the high-GI category.

Table 5.1: High-GI Foods and Low-GI Foods

High-GI Foods

Sugar – table sugar, high-fructose corn syrup, milk chocolate, sweets, etc.
All wheat breads – white bread and brown bread
White rice
White pasta
Potatoes
Breakfast cereals
Jams, syrups, marmalades and jellies
Sweetened drinks
Alcohol

Low-GI Foods

Natural sweeteners – stevia and xylitol
Dark chocolate
Non-wheat breads
Oats – flakes or oat cakes
Legumes – lentils, peas and beans
Fruit and vegetables

Tea – rooibos and green tea

Meat – beef, lamb, pork, chicken and turkey

Brown rice

Brown pasta

I would go so far as to say that you should not eat too many of the low-GI foods either. If you do choose to use a form of starch to boost your energy levels, choose it from the low-GI category, but do not make starchy foods the core of your diet. Government advice in the form of the food pyramid is to eat many servings of starch a day; in other words, to make starch the principal food for every meal. This not only ignores scientific research but actively promotes obesity and, worse still, cancer.

Rather than informing people that if they want to prevent cancer they should avoid all sugar and wheat flour, as well as commercial breakfast cereals and the other foods that have a high glycaemic index, drug companies are now searching for drugs that will lower insulin and IGF levels. Their motivation is profit, not your well-being. They are quite content to let you poison your body with high levels of sugar.

Dairy Produce

Years ago I remember reading an article about the use of the pesticide lindane and its association with breast cancer. In those days dairy herds were dusted with this pesticide to kill pests on the skin. The pesticide was absorbed through the skin of the animal and trace amounts were found in the milk. Because there was a reported association between exposure to lindane and breast cancer, two countries,

Finland and Israel, banned the use of it. The incidence of breast cancer dropped in both of these countries.

The use of chemicals, hormone treatments, drugs and so on in modern farming knows no limits. Despite a wealth of evidence that we are doing serious harm to the environment and to farm animals, and indeed to ourselves, the use of these substances continues.

As I mentioned in Chapter 3, there is now growing evidence that the major protein in milk, casein, is a promoter of cancer. In *The China Study*, it is described it as a category 1 carcinogen (Campbell and Campbell, 2006). In other words, it fulfills all of the criteria established by the IARC, part of the World Health Organization, to be a carcinogen.

This startling information is hard to believe, but the research is very convincing. However, is dairy the problem in itself? If so, the Maasai in East Africa and the Fulani in West Africa, both of whom herd cattle and depend on a supply of raw milk every day as their main source of food, would show evidence of a high incidence of cancer. Rather, the incidence of cancer among them is close to zero. How can this be explained?

The only plausible explanation is that the process of pasteurisation is making the milk toxic. Pasteurisation exposes milk to high temperatures for a short time. It is known that heat damages protein and can render it harmful. Pasteurisation also kills all the good bacteria in the milk and destroys the enzymes, making it much more difficult to digest. I suspect that this is the reason why more and more people are becoming intolerant to milk.

But can it be possible that milk and dairy products are bad for us? Many of us were brought up to believe that milk is good for us. We were taught that the calcium in milk is essential for strong bones and teeth and that it is important to eat cheese if you have osteoporosis or osteopaenia. Well, evidence from many sources confirms that milk does indeed contain cancer-causing substances.

Pasteurised milk has been shown to contain a cocktail of hormones and growth factors. It has been shown to have as many as thirty-five different hormones and eleven different growth factors, some of which are known to promote the growth and the spread of cancer. For example, high levels of IGF and an even more dangerous growth factor, vascular endothelial growth factor (VEGF), have been found in dairy produce (Azzouz *et al.*, 2011).

If this theory that milk can cause cancer is correct, then people who abstain from milk, such as vegans, should have a lower incidence of cancer compared to those who drink milk. A study performed by Oxford University scientists showed that the level of IGF was significantly lower in vegans compared to vegetarians and meat eaters. This research was reported in the *Journal of Cancer Research* (Allen *et al.*, 2000). Two years later, another research study was reported in a different cancer research journal, which confirmed that IGF levels were indeed lower in vegans (Allen *et al.*, 2002). This evidence confirms that the consumption of cow's milk is indeed a serious issue. This is not a suggestion or a supposition; it is firmly rooted in hard scientific data that consuming pasteurised milk increases your risk of cancer.

We should take this evidence seriously, and if we wish to avoid cancer we should exclude all commercial dairy produce from our diet, or at least reduce it to a minimum.

Personally, I believe that raw milk is safe to drink, provided it has been tested for brucellosis and tuberculosis. I do not have scientific evidence to confirm this, but from looking at the evidence of the Maasai and Fulani tribes in Africa, and the lower instances of cancer historically when people drank unpasteurised milk, I believe that pasteurisation rather than milk itself is the problem.

––––––

You can now better appreciate how the typical Western diet feeds cancer and why the incidence of cancer in countries that follow a Western diet has increased since the 1940s. As mentioned, during the Second World War, when there was food rationing, the use of cheap foods such as sugar and white flour increased. This pattern has increased despite the end of rationing in the 1950s. Then, in 1974, there was another major shift in the Western food production: the removal or reduction of saturated fat in a range of foods and the replacement of this fat with sugar. This may well explain the increase in many cancers since the mid-1970s.

There is little doubt that a number of foods in the modern diet are acting as promoters of cancer. I have mentioned sugar, wheat, dairy and artificial sweeteners. The next food that I want to look at is margarine.

Margarine
In the 1950s another factor came into play that altered the Western diet for the worse and further predisposed the population to cancer. It was the belief that animal fat causes heart disease, which we all now know is totally false.

Because of the belief that animal fat is harmful, we were sold the idea that vegetable oils and margarine are much safer. Along came names such as Flora margarine and various brands of low-fat spread, which exploited this and made so much profit that they were able to sponsor national heart foundations and sports events, etc. To the present day, doctors still advise patients who have high cholesterol or heart disease to cut down on eggs, butter, cheese and so on. Yet there is not a scrap of hard scientific evidence linking dietary fat and heart disease.

Many of the commercial spreads and margarines contain trans fats, which are very harmful and are known to cause such serious health problems that certain governments have banned them, for example the Dutch government. These margarines or vegetable oil spreads are manufactured using tiny particles of nickel and aluminium. Some of these metal particles end up in the finished product and then you consume them. Nickel is carcinogenic and aluminium is implicated in Alzheimer's disease (Nordberg, 2007).

These margarines also affect your immune system by reducing the effectiveness of certain immune responses; for example, they impair the ability of your immune system to make antibodies. These spreads also interfere with the liver's ability to metabolise toxins and carcinogens, making you more susceptible to cancer (Erasmus, 1993).

The main reason why some governments have banned them is because they are hormone disrupters. They can therefore interfere with pregnancy and reduce the quality of breast milk. As disrupters of the hormonal system they can presdispose to hormone-based cancers such as breast cancer in women and prostate cancer in men.

If you do have to use these spreads for whatever reason, use them sparingly; better still, avoid them completely. They are yet another attempt by industry to pull the wool over your eyes.

The aim when eating fats is to get the balance of omega 6 as close to omega 3 as possible. Vegetable oil spreads and margarines are rich in omega 6 but devoid of any omega 3. This in itself is not a bad thing as long as you take an equivalent amount of omega 3 as fish oil or flaxseed oil. Because of the manufacturing process, the omega 6 in spreads and margarines become pro-inflammatory and as you now know, chronic consumption of foods that promote inflammation also promote cancer.

As discussed in Chapter 3, in the good old days, free range eggs had equal amount of omega 6 and omega 3. Nowadays, most eggs have a high amount of omega 6 and little or no omega 3. This is true of most fat-containing foods in the modern diet. That's why there is so much advice suggesting a greater consumption of omega 3. This is why fish oils and flaxseed have become very popular supplements for people to take.

————

Many of the people who come to *see* me in my clinic have had blood tests or an upper scope (gastroscopy) done and have been declared free of coeliac disease; yet they still have gut symptoms. On further testing, I find that many of them are reacting negatively to either gluten or dairy, or in some cases to both of these.

It's easy to *see* why a number of my patients end up on restrictive diets, especially diets excluding the three big role players in ill health – sugar, gluten and dairy. All three, in addition to causing inflammation in the gut, can also promote the growth and spread of cancer.

If you want to do yourself a big favour, go on a sugar-free, gluten-free and dairy-free diet for a period of time, say one month, and notice improvements in your overall health. There are recipe books that can help with this. One of the best is *The Extra Virgin Kitchen* by Susan Jane White (Gill & Macmillan, 2014).

FOODS TO INCLUDE IN YOUR DIET

The immense power of diet to influence cancer in a positive way was demonstrated by Professor Dean Ornish of the University of California. He showed that prostate cancer could be reversed by diet alone. His research showed that diet had a powerful effect on which genes got switched on and which were switched off. In other words, it demonstrated conclusively in the form of a randomised, controlled clinical trial how certain foods were able to influence the epigenome and so restore the cells back to health. The diet that Dr Ornish used in this clinical trial was a vegan diet. It was reported in the journal *Proceedings of the National Academy of Sciences* (Ornish *et al.*, 2008).

A short period of three months on such a diet had the effect of switching off 450 cancer genes and switching on 48 protective genes in patients. This is excellent news for anyone who has cancer and even better news for anyone who wishes to avoid cancer. Now, let's examine some of the elements of the diet that offers protection against cancer.

Green Tea

Surely there must be more important aspects of a protective diet, I hear you say. Surely we are not going to stoop to the level of discussing tea. Well, believe it or not, the kind of tea you drink has a significant effect on your health. For more than a decade it has been known that green tea can protect against cancer.

Green tea is thought to be one of the reasons why there is a low lung cancer incidence among Chinese who smoke a lot compared to Westerners who also smoke cigarettes. Could green tea actually protect the body against the carcinogens in cigarette smoke? Green tea has attracted a lot of interest from scientists and doctors over the past decade and research on it has indeed shown that it acts as an antioxidant. It *see*ms to activate chemical reactions in the liver to allow the detoxification and removal of harmful carcinogens. It acts in a similar way to vitamin C but appears to be even more potent (Jankun *et al.*, 1997).

According to the National Cancer Institute in the USA, green tea contains certain antioxidant substances called catechins. One of these substances has been shown to block the formation of new blood vessels by cancer cells, hence starving the cells of food and oxygen. By doing so, it prevents the local invasion of a cancer into healthy neighbouring tissue and so halts local spread (Demeule *et al.*, 2005).

In his research, Professor Béliveau tested the effectiveness of the active ingredient in green tea on several types of cancer cells. His research confirmed the fact that this substance was able to significantly slow the growth of a number of cancers, including breast cancer, prostate cancer and leukaemia, as well as skin cancer and kidney cancer (Béliveau and Gingas, 2006).

For those who already have cancer there is also great benefit to drinking green tea. Green tea, as is the case with many other protective foods, seems to enhance the therapeutic benefit of both chemotherapy and radiotherapy. It seems to make the cancer cells more sensitive to conventional medical anti-cancer treatment, often meaning that lower doses of radiotherapy, for example, can be used, thus lessening the damage done to healthy tissue (McLaughlin, 2006).

Protective foods such as green tea all seem to have synergistic properties, in that when they are combined in the diet the benefits are greater than when each is taken separately. The Laboratory of Nutrition and Metabolism at Harvard Medical School showed that when green tea is combined with soya in the diet, this combination works better than when each is taken separately (Zhou, 2004). In other words, if you add to your diet all of the protective foods I am going to mention in the next few pages, their beneficial effect will be enhanced significantly.

The authors of the Harvard Medical School study suggest in their research paper that soya and green tea may form an effective dietary regimen for inhibiting the progression of oestrogen-dependent tumours, especially breast cancer. This is quite a statement from a very conservative medical establishment.

Classically, green tea has been associated with China where it is drunk widely throughout the country. However, Japanese green tea is even richer in all the catechins and so is even better to use if you can source it. When making the tea, allow it to brew for five minutes for the active ingredients to be released. Drink as many cups a day as you can; the more the better. Green tea contains caffeine; however, if it upsets your system, I would not recommend the use of the decaffeinated version as its production involves the addition of the dangerous industrial chemical trichloroethylene.

When purchasing green tea, try to buy organic brands as lots of chemical sprays – the same fertilisers and sprays used on wheat and barley – are used in growing most tea and coffee plants. These are nitrogen fertilisers, which speed up the growth of the plant but weaken it, making it more vulnerable to disease. Therefore, fungicides are used to control fungal infections, insecticides are used to tackle insect invasions and weedkillers such as Roundup are used to prevent weeds. These chemicals are extremely toxic to humans.

A group of Canadian doctors was so concerned about people being exposed to a cocktail of chemicals day after day, year after year, that they decided to review a lot of the research done to date. The Ontario College of Family Physicians' study, which was published in April 2012, found definite links between pesticide exposure and various health problems. Among these problems were damage to the central nervous system, respiratory problems such as asthma, and a whole range of reproductive and fertility issues in both sexes. This isn't surprising as some of these chemicals, such as the insecticide Malathion, are known toxins and carcinogens (Ontario College of Family Physicians, 2012).

Rooibos Tea

This tea plant originates from Southern Africa and the Cape Province of South Africa in particular. This is quite a different plant from green tea and so has a different array of beneficial chemicals. In particular, it contains quercetin and luteolin, both of which have been shown to have both anti-cancer and anti-inflammatory effects (Rubin, 2010; Marnewick et al., 2009). This effectively makes rooibos tea an excellent anti-cancer substance.

Rooibos tea is rich in antioxidants, especially vitamin C, which is one of the main reasons why it has become so popular, not just in southern Africa but across the world. Most of the major companies that sell ordinary black tea now include rooibos tea as one of their products. This is mainly due to the proven health benefits of rooibos and its consequent growing popularity (Theunissen, 2005).

In 2011, researchers carried out a clinical trial to test the benefits of drinking rooibos tea. They looked at the risk factors for heart disease such as raised LDL cholesterol, low HDL cholesterol, lipid peroxidation and so on. Those people who drank significant amounts of rooibos tea were shown to have lower levels of these risk factors than those who did not (Marnewick et al., 2011). This clearly indicates the health benefits of this remarkable plant.

The nice thing about rooibos tea is that it looks like and tastes like ordinary black tea but it has no caffeine and a much lower level of tannin. If you don't like herbal teas or green tea, then try rooibos: it can improve your health and protect against cancer.

Turmeric

This is a spice that is used widely in Indian cooking. However, it is also widely used in Ayurvedic medicine, the oldest form of medicine, as an anti-inflammatory. One of the main researchers to demonstrate the amazing benefits of this spice is Professor Bharat Aggarwal, who is a very eminent researcher at the MD Anderson Cancer Center in Houston, Texas. He was born and brought up in Punjab, India where he first learned of the amazing properties of this plant. When he was asked to do research on experimental cancer therapies, he used his knowledge of Ayurveda to help in this task. It is thanks to him that we now have hard scientific data supporting turmeric as an anti-cancer substance.

In Chapter 3, I discussed the role of inflammation in the growth and spread of cancer. Professor Aggarwal demonstrated the role of certain factors in generating inflammation and showed that one factor in particular plays a major role in both the growth of cancer and its spread. This pro-inflammatory factor is secreted by cancer cells and ensures a steady supply of nutrients to the cells. We saw in Chapter 3 that this factor is referred to as nuclear factor or, to give it its full title, nuclear factor kappa B.

In 2004, the journal *Science* published an article dealing with the role of pro-inflammatory factors in cancer growth and development. It concluded that not only was nuclear factor the most important but that almost every cancer preventive is an inhibitor of it (Marx, 2004). The whole of the drug industry is searching for a drug that will effectively inhibit nuclear factor. However, there are many natural substances that already do this very effectively. One of them is turmeric.

There is no other plant or food substance with the same powerful anti-inflammatory properties as turmeric. The principal active ingredient in turmeric is a molecule called **curcumin.** In many studies on laboratory animals it has been shown to inhibit the growth of a large number of cancers. For example, it has been shown to protect against human breast cancer (Mehta *et al.,* 1997).

What is even more interesting is the fact that it blocks the initial development of primary tumours after the body has been exposed to known carcinogens. So, even if you are at risk of getting cancer because you have smoked heavily, for example, turmeric can act a protector (Cheng *et al.,* 2001). It is no wonder that it's so highly regarded by Ayurvedic medicine.

Indians eat a lot of turmeric. This may explain why cancer incidence is so low in India compared to the West. Cancer of the colon, for example, is approximately 10 per cent of what it is in the West. The statistics for other cancers are also very low in India and indeed in the whole of Asia.

Professor Aggarwal was the first to show that curcumin, the active ingredient in turmeric, is active against cancer cell cultures. In 2005 he demonstrated that curcumin was active in killing breast cancer cells grafted onto mice. The mice were fed curcumin in their food and monitored for the development of secondary tumours. Curcumin efficiently blocked the spread of cancer in these mice. In other words, curcumin was able to inhibit the dark knight of cancer, the pro-inflammatory nuclear factor (Aggarwal *et al.,* 2005).

If you wish to add lots of turmeric to your meals, it is worthwhile being aware that turmeric is not well absorbed across the gut wall. However, black pepper helps its absorption, so it's good to take the two at the same time. In that way you will get the benefit of one of the best anti-cancer foods available.

Soya

In many schools across China children are given soya milk instead of cow's milk at break time. The Chinese, Japanese and many other Asian people have been using soya in their diet for thousands of years. For the past two thousand years the Chinese have regarded it as one of the five sacred foods. It is now thought that this is one of the reasons why China has one of the lowest rates of hormone-based cancers in the world.

Figure 5.1: Incidence of Breast Cancer among Chinese Who Live in USA Compared to Those Who Live in China

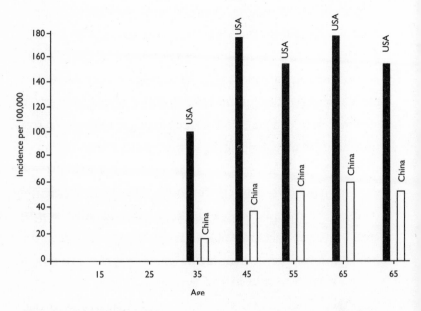

Source: Servan-Schreiber, D., *Anticancer: A New Way of Life*, London: Michael Joseph, 2011: 73.

As mentioned, once Chinese people move away from China and/or adopt a Western diet they begin to show up with more breast cancer, prostate cancer and other hormone-based cancers. Figure 5.1 demonstrates this in the case of breast cancer. In addition, in the past ten years breast cancer rates in the main cities of China, where many people consume a Western diet, have tripled. The same rapid increase is *see*n in Japanese and Chinese immigrants to Europe and North America.

The main benefit of consuming soya is that it contains plant oestrogens (phytoestrogens) that block other harmful forms of oestrogen. When any form of oestrogen attaches to the receptor of a breast cell it can alter the chemistry of the cell, which can result in certain cancer genes being switched on and protective genes being switched off. This is shown in Figure 5.2.

Figure 5.2: *Effect of Oestrogen on a Breast Cell*

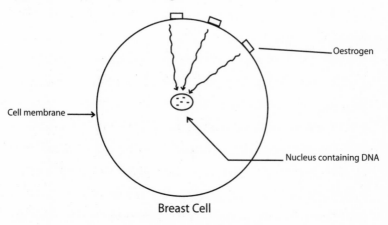

Breast Cell

Oestrogen has a strong effect on DNA.

Any form of oestrogen, including oestrogen in the contraceptive pill, hormone replacement therapy (HRT), water and food, including soya, will attach to the cells in the body that are influenced by oestrogen or have oestrogen receptors. What separates soya oestrogen from all other forms is that its effects on the cell are so minimal that it is not regarded as a disrupter of the hormonal system; rather, it is viewed as a protector of the hormonal system because it prevents other harmful forms of oestrogen from attaching to the cell receptor sites, so nullifying their negative effects.

Figure 5.3 compares the effects of oestrogen in soya and oestrogen in the contraceptive pill. As you can *see*, the effect of soya oestrogen is minimal, whereas that of oestrogen in the pill is much more pronounced.

If you wish to learn more about where oestrogen is found in your environment, read the section entitled 'Oestrogen and Other Hormone Disrupters in Your Environment' in Chapter 2.

So, soya is a really good food to add to your diet, either as the raw plant or milk, or in its fermented form. In combination with other anti-cancer foods, it offers excellent protection, especially if you are being exposed to oestrogen in your drinking water or from foods wrapped in plastic, or if you are being exposed to high levels of oestrogen produced by stored fat in the body.

The one main disadvantage associated with soya is that it is quite allergenic. It ranks high up the list of foods that people commonly react to. If you can tolerate it well all the better, but if you can't, use another form of milk such as goat, sheep or buffalo milk, or rice, almond or coconut milk.

Figure 5.3: Effects of Soya and the Contraceptive Pill on a Breast Cell

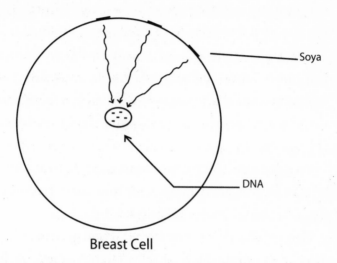

Breast Cell

Soya has a weak effect on DNA – minimal chemical disturbance.

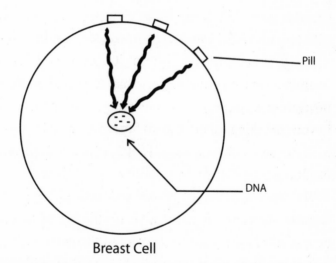

Breast Cell

The pill has a strong effect on DNA – maximal chemical disturbance.

Omega 3 Oils

On a basic level, we can view omega 3 oils – fish oil and flaxseed oil – as anti-inflammatory and therefore anti-cancer, and omega 6 oils – corn oil, rapeseed oil, sunflower oil – as pro-inflammatory and pro-cancer. However, as discussed in Chapter 3, we should be eating a balanced intake of these oils, but in a typical Western diet this is far from the case.

I used to test omega 6 and omega 3 levels in new patients, but after a while I had to give up as the results were always the same – too much omega 6 and a deficiency of omega 3. Nowadays, I just assume everyone is omega 3 deficient and act accordingly.

People's diets simply no longer contain sufficient levels of omega 3. This has to do with the way animals such as hens are raised and fed today (*see* Chapter 3).

This same imbalance of too much omega 6 to omega 3 in eggs occurs in the milk of dairy herds that are not fed on natural grasslands but on cattle feed containing cereals such as soya and corn. Table 5.2 compares the ratio of omega 6 to omega 3 in different foods in 1950 and 2010.

Table 5.2: *The Ratio of Omega 6 to Omega 3 in Different Foods in 1950 and 2010*

Foods	1950	2010
Butter	3:1	7:1
Beef	4:1	16:1
Eggs	3:1	30:1

Source: Hibbeln, J. *et al.*, 'Quantitative changes in the availability of fats in the US food supply', 5th Congress of the International Society for the Study of Fatty Acids and Lipids, Montreal, 7–11 May 2002: 10.

As you can *see* from Table 5.2, the levels of omega 6 have risen significantly over the years from 1950 to 2000. We are now consuming much more omega 6, which has two main effects: to promote inflammation and stimulate cell growth. The level of omega 3 in our diet has dropped, yet this is a protective oil as it is anti-inflammatory and controls cell growth.

If using eggs or meat, use organic, free-range eggs and meat from grass-fed animals. Also, take flax*seed* oil or fish oil daily to boost your levels of the protective omega 3. In this way your body will be better able to control inflammation and cell growth, both factors in the development of cancer.

In addition, make sure that your diet contains an essential oil called conjugated linoleic acid (CLA). In even small amounts, it has been proven to have strong anti-cancer properties (Harvey, 2008). It is found only in grass-fed animals such as goats, sheep and cattle. Milk from organic-ally raised animals has even higher levels of nutrients such as CLA.

Mushrooms

In a number of hospitals in Japan, mushrooms are given to cancer patients for therapeutic reasons. For example, research has shown better survival rates for patients with colon cancer who are given mushrooms during or after chemotherapy (Kidd, 2000).

The most commonly used mushrooms that are beneficial are shiitake, maitake, kawaratake and enokitake mushrooms. These mushrooms are used extensively in Japanese cooking. They have been tested scientifically and found to have powerful immunity-enhancing properties. They *see*m to act by stimulating natural killer cells, which are an integral part of the immune system (Kidd, 2000). Research has shown that the consumption of these mushrooms leads to an increase in both the number of natural killer cells as well as the activity of these cells, making them an ideal food for anyone with cancer or to prevent cancer. Japanese peasants who consume a lot of these mushrooms have a 50 per cent lower rate of stomach cancer compared to those who don't (Hara *et al.*, 2003).

Professor Béliveau has tested many types of mushroom on cancer cells and produced some very exciting results. Some of the mushrooms showed definite benefit, in combating breast cancer cells in particular. He tried the Japanese mushrooms mentioned above but discovered that oyster mushrooms and thistle oyster mushrooms were the most effective in stopping the growth of cancer cells (Béliveau and Gingas, 2006).

My advice is to start adding therapeutic mushrooms to your diet and consume them frequently. Never pick them from the wild – it can be hard to tell the difference between edible mushrooms and poisonous types – but rather buy them from a vegetable shop or health food shop.

Berries

Nearly all berries show anti-cancer properties. Many of these berries have been tested by Professor Béliveau, who has discovered the ways in which they prevent cancer. In testing foods for anti-cancer properties, he first tested them on cancer cells in test tubes to *see* if they could control the growth rate of the cancer. Those foods that showed they had anti-cancer properties were then tested on laboratory animals. In addition, he isolated the active ingredients in the foods and subjected these to testing. In this way, it was possible for him to determine why certain foods are effective at controlling the growth of cancers.

He tested a range of fruits and found that certain berries had definite anti-cancer properties. Raspberries and strawberries in particular showed a lot of promise. He showed that these berries have the effect of blocking the growth of new blood vessels necessary for the growth and spread of cancer cells. The berries *seem* to block two very important growth factors that are known to stimulate the growth of new blood vessels (Béliveau and Gingas, 2006).

Drug companies would pay millions for the discovery of a drug that could do this. In fact, they already have. In 2004, a drug that works against cancer in a very similar way to raspberries was released under the trade name Avastin. Like raspberries, it blocks one of the growth factors involved in stimulating the growth of new capillaries.

Professor Béliveau isolated the active ingredient in raspberries as ellagic acid and discovered that not only does this substance have anti-cancer properties if cancer has already developed, but it protects the body against the development of cancer in the first place. It blocks harmful carcinogens from doing damage in the body, i.e. the *seed* stage of cancer development. In other words, it helps the liver to detoxify carcinogenic substances and eliminate them from the body. Therefore, these berries *seem* to help the body in a variety of ways and are not limited to one mode of action as many drugs are, such as Avastin.

Ellagic acid is found in large amounts in strawberries,

raspberries and pomegranates, as well as in nuts such as hazelnuts and walnuts. It has been extensively researched using cell cultures and animal studies and does indeed *seem* to have anti-cancer actions. One of the few studies of this compound involving humans was carried out in Italy, where it was shown to reduce the side effects of chemotherapy in patients with prostate cancer (Falsaperla *et al.*, 2005). Many more studies on humans need to be done to confirm the positive effects of this substance.

However, in addition to strawberries and raspberries, many other berries have been shown to have anti-cancer actions. Some berries, such as blueberries and cranberries, contain substances that can force cancer cells to die. These compounds are called anthocyanidins and proantho-cyanidins. The same compounds are found in dark chocolate.

A product that I use every morning is called Seeds for Cereal and is manufactured by Virginia Harvest in west Cork, Ireland. It contains blueberries and cranberries combined with milled flax*seed*, making it one of the best combination products if you want to stay healthy and reduce your risk of getting cancer.

Garlic, Onions and Shallots

It is no accident that most soups, stir-fries and stews have a basis of garlic and onions fried in oil. Garlic and onions or shallots are the first ingredients in many naturally prepared meals.

These are foods that are rich in sulphur and so help the liver to detoxify harmful chemicals. They are also strongly antibacterial and prevent infection while keeping the bacterial flora intact. Because they can control infections, they are important in the regulation of cancers that are associated with certain infections.

Table 5.3 lists the chronic infections in the body that can ultimately lead to cancer. Probably the best known of these is the human papillomavirus (HPV), which is an infection of the cervix and can lead to the development of cervical cancer.

Another well-known association is the chronic infection of the stomach wall with *Helicobacter pylori* and stomach cancer. One of the reasons why stomach cancer has actually declined in the West is because many more people are being treated for this infection.

Table 5.3: Chronic Infections that Can Lead to Cancer

Chronic Infections	Associated Cancer
Hepatitis	Primary liver cancer
Helicobacter pylori	Stomach cancer
Human papillomavirus	Cervical cancer
Bilharzia	Bladder cancer
Herpes virus type 8	Kaposi sarcoma

Garlic and onions are not only antibacterial but can also stabilise the blood sugar levels. This in turn reduces insulin release and thus reduces the secretion of the growth factor IGF.

Therefore, eat lots of garlic, onion and shallots, either raw in salads or cooked in soups and stir-fries. They will help your liver function, prevent a rise in blood sugar levels and help control infections. They are the most important ingredients in almost any meal.

Vegetables and Fruit

All the brightly coloured vegetables and fruits, such as tomatoes, peppers, carrots and so on, are important anti-cancer agents. They all contain vitamin A and lycopene, both of which have been shown to inhibit the growth of a number of different types of cancer.

Lycopene has the effect of stimulating the activity of the immune system, especially that of natural killer cells, a type of white blood cell that can attack and destroy cancer cells. We saw in Chapter 1 that Mighty Mouse had very active natural killer cells, which were able to fight off cancer cells even after the cancer had taken hold. Regardless of the dosage of cancer cells injected into the mouse, it was able to mobilise its immune system to fight back and win.

Much research on the antioxidants in vegetables and fruit has been done in the laboratory in animal testing. Therefore, it can be hard to make definitive statements about these studies in the case of humans. However, one very interesting study followed breast cancer patients over a six-year period to *see* if brightly coloured fruit and vegetables made any difference to their survival rate. The study showed that those patients who consumed more fruit and vegetables actually lived significantly longer (Ingram *et al.*, 1994).

Eating lots of vegetables and fruit has a number of health benefits, and research shows that cancer prevention may be one of them. One of the reasons why the cancer rate is so low in Asia could be that the Asian diet is based on vegetables and fruit.

SUMMARY

It is becoming more apparent from scientific and medical research that diet plays a key role in both causing and preventing cancer. The single most significant culprit in causing cancer is sugar. Over the past century, but especially in the last thirty years, the consumption of sugar in the Western world has skyrocketed. Everyone who consumes a Western diet has been subjected to more and more sugar hidden in processed foods.

As I discussed in this chapter, sugar is linked directly with the promotion and spread of cancer. It supplies cancer cells with food, allowing them to thrive and multiply. Sugar has other hidden dangers as well. It blocks the therapeutic benefit of anti-cancer substances and drugs. For example, it reduces the effectiveness of chemotherapy on a range of cancer cells. It makes it much harder for the body to fight off cancer.

The problem is that sugar is highly addictive and is hard to cut out of the diet. When I ask some of my patients to remove sugar from their diet, they are often shocked at how many foods and drinks contain sugar. They are also shocked at how difficult it is to give up.

It's not just sugar that is a danger in the Western diet. Any food that raises blood sugar levels – high-GI foods (wheat, white rice, potatoes, etc.), for example, can be a problem as well. Like sugar, these foods can promote the growth and spread of cancer. It is best to keep them to a minimum or avoid them completely.

Since the publication of Professor Campbell's research suggesting that milk protein – casein – is a definite promoter of cancer, the sales of milk and milk products (cheese, yoghurt, etc.) have dropped. His work has prompted a change in the perception of what constitutes a healthy diet, not least on the part of Harvard University.

Butter is a much healthier food than vegetable oil spreads as the latter contain trans fats, which are harmful. Butter is of course a dairy product, but it does not contain the protein casein; it contains the fat portion of milk. Use organic butter, which is available in most good supermarkets.

However, healthy eating and anti-cancer diets are not just about avoiding harmful foods; they're also about eating foods that have a proven ability to counteract cancer. These anti-cancer foods include herbs, spices and teas, which are often overlooked by dieticians, nutritionists and doctors when they are advising patients. One may be forgiven for not classifying spices, herbs and teas as providing important nutrients, but they *seem* to be important, if you trust the research.

During his time at the University of Montreal, Professor Béliveau documented the anti-cancer properties of a range of foods. From laboratory experiments, he has drawn up a list of beneficial foods with proven anti-cancer effects. These foods include green tea, turmeric, soya, mushrooms, berries, and many fruits and vegetables. His work is truly ground-breaking.

Chapter 6
How to Change Your Diet

Having read the previous chapters, you may feel ready to make adjustments to your eating habits. It's quite easy to do this provided you abandon what I refer to as 'the herd mentality'. You must have the courage to abandon old beliefs, and be prepared to swim upstream and to challenge the norm. In other words, you have to think and act differently from the rest of the society. For a society to change it takes about 20 per cent of the population, the pioneers, to make that change and then the rest of society will follow suit.

You may have experienced cancer among the people in your community, or closer to home, within your family, or you may have had cancer in the past. These experiences are important motivations to learn and make the necessary changes to your diet and lifestyle.

It's worth regarding change as an evolutionary process. It does not happen overnight and it requires time and patience. Introduce the changes to your diet at a pace that suits you and your family. Be kind to yourself and don't get frustrated if you cannot find a particular food item in your local shops.

You can try to delete foods from your diet gradually and introduce new foods.

Having treated people using restrictive diets for the past thirty years, I know that this is not easy and that it requires determination. It is also quite anti-social as you will require foods that are not readily available in restaurants or at events. I generally say to people that as long as they follow treatment 90 per cent of the time, healing will take place; if you have to attend a party or wedding or other event, go with the flow and take small amounts of the potentially harmful foodstuffs.

Your taste buds will change when you follow a new diet. You will slowly lose the craving for certain foods, such as sweets, desserts, salty products and so on. You will also begin to appreciate the taste of fresh healthy foods. As you stick to a healthy, more natural diet, your body will show the signs of healing and often other people will comment on how well you look even before you notice it.

Below, I suggest possible steps to help make the transition from an unhealthy diet to a much healthier one easier.

THE STEPS TO A HEALTHY DIET
Step 1
The first and most important food to exclude from the diet is dairy produce – cheese, milk, yoghurt, cream and ice-cream. Dairy is everywhere in the modern world and most people are not aware of the damage it is causing (*see* Chapters 3 and 5). It is an allergenic food, it promotes the growth of cancer cells, and many harmful chemicals used by farmers can be found in the fat content, including hormones to encourage more milk production by the cow. It is a highly commercial product and so should be regarded as susceptible to political interference.

Instead of dairy, use organic soya milk products or one of the other milk products now becoming more available, such as buffalo milk, almond milk and rice milk (should be free from arsenic). Alternatively, if you are not allergic to dairy and the cattle have been raised organically then it should be possible to continue to use non-commercial dairy produce, such as raw unpasteurised milk and raw milk products –yoghurt, butter, cheese, etc.

Step 2

Remove sugar from your diet as much as possible. It is very difficult to exclude sugar completely as almost every processed food has some sugar and even many so-called healthier products, such as energy bars and energy drinks, also contain sugar.

Get yourself into the habit of reading food labels, though admittedly these can be very confusing. To determine the level of sugar in a product, look at the table entitled 'Nutritional Information'. This table will tell you what percentage of the product is composed of carbohydrate and immediately underneath it will say, 'of which sugars are'. This will give the percentage of sugar in 100 grams of the food item, as shown in Figure 6.1.

The next thing to examine on a food label is the list of ingredients so that you can *see* which sugars have been used. Be careful with the following sugars: sucrose, table sugar, corn syrup, high fructose corn syrup, inverted (or invert) sugar, fructose and glucose. Also check to *see* if any artificial sweeteners have been used – sucralose, aspartame, acesulfame K or saccharin – and don't buy the product if these have been included.

Figure 6.1: Nutritional Information Table

NUTRITIONAL INFORMATION		
Typical Values	Per Biscuit	Per 100g
Energy	183kj	1830kj
	44kcal	436kcal
Protein	0.7g	7.4g
Available Carbohydrate	6.4g	63.7g
of which sugars	2.2g	21.7g
Fat	1.7g	16.8g
of which saturates	0.7g	7.5g
Fibre	0.6g	5.6g
Salt	0.04g	0.40g
Sodium	0.03g	0.29g
GUIDELINE DAILY AMOUNTS		
	Women	Men
Calories	2000kcal	2500kcal
Fat	70g	95g
Salt	6g	6g

Buy products that contain natural sweeteners (for example, honey or maple syrup) instead of sugar or artificial sweeteners, and if cooking or baking use natural substances such as stevia or xylitol. These are now readily available in most supermarkets.

Step 3

If you have managed to exclude dairy and sugar and are using safer alternatives, then you are well ahead. Cancer needs sugar to grow and needs promoters such as casein, the protein in milk. Because wheat is known as a high-GI food (foods that stimulate the release of insulin and the growth factor IGF, which is implicated in stimulating the growth of cancer cells), it would be best to reduce the wheat in your diet to a minimum.

Instead of wheat-based breads, cereals and pasta, use gluten-free options such as foods made from corn, buckwheat and quinoa. It is still possible to eat breakfast cereal, bread and pasta as long as they are made using a gluten-free cereal. Spelt is another option. It is not gluten free, but it contains less gluten than wheat. In most health shops it is possible to buy spelt flakes or muesli, spelt flour, spelt breads and spelt pasta. These are much safer options and are better able to protect you against cancer.

Step 4

Do not use processed meats, especially meats from the deli section of your supermarket – pepperoni, salami and so on. If you want to use chicken, beef or pork, try to get organic meat from your local butcher or farmers' market. The fat content of meat and meat products can be quite toxic as this is where a lot of the agricultural chemicals that the animal may have been exposed to are stored.

Add garlic and onions to each meal, especially soups, stews and stir-fries. Garlic and onions have anti-cancer properties, as discussed in Chapter 5. Also, turmeric, in particular, has been proven to have significant anti-cancer effects, and would be a healthy addition to a meat dish or any cooked meal.

Step 5

Change from ordinary black tea to green tea. Green tea can be an acquired taste, so do persist if at first you don't like it. Buy organic tea leaves rather than tea bags, but if you can't source the leaves, begin with bags. Allow the tea to stand for a while, say five minutes, to allow the catechins (the active ingredients) to be released. Drink at least 2–3 cups a day. If you don't like the taste, switch to rooibos tea. Suppliers of rooibos tea include Rooibos Ireland, Millicant House, Lower Dargle Road, Bray, County Wicklow (email owenb dawson@eircom.net), and one supplier of green tea is Clipper Teas Ltd, Beaminster, Dorset, DT8 3PR, England.

Reduce your coffee intake to a minimum as coffee has been associated with bladder cancer. Although the IARC has listed coffee as a possible carcinogen, there is some evidence that it may actually protect against certain cancers – oral cancers, cancer of the pharynx and oesophageal cancer. Despite these reported benefits, I would still advise you to reduce your coffee intake as coffee stimulates the release of stress hormones – adrenalin and cortisol. So an occasional cup of coffee is fine, as long as you get your caffeine from green tea most of the time.

Step 6

Become a mushroom expert. Learn about different types of mushroom and add them to salads, omelettes, stews and stir-fries. When frying them, use butter instead of cooking oil. Mushrooms are a tasty addition to any meal, and because they have such a positive effect on immunity they can be a real bonus in keeping cancer at bay (*see* Chapter 5).

Due to the high levels of arsenic in most forms of rice (*see* Chapter 2), it is best to exclude rice from your diet as much as possible. Some forms of basmati rice are safer, but both white and wholegrain rice are problematic. Also, do not buy rice products for young children, such as rice cereal, rice pudding, rice milk.

Step 7

Become much more aware of the foods you are eating and the drinks you consume, and make a habit of reading food and drink labels. It is only by learning more that you'll be able to clean up your diet and supply your body with what it really needs to function in your best interests.

I am now going to discuss the key components of a healthy diet so that you have a global idea of what your body needs.

THE COMPONENTS OF A HEALTHY DIET

Healthy foods correspond to what the body is composed of. A body composition analyser is a really useful device that doctors can use to determine where you are at nutritionally. It tells you what percentage of your body is water, what percentage is fat, what percentage is protein and so on. It also determines your body mass index (a measure of your body fat using your height and weight) and therefore can indicate if you are overweight, underweight or normal; it also compares your biological age with your chronological age.

Water

I looked at water in detail in Chapter 3. Since we are composed of about 50 to 60 per cent water, it is worth getting the quality of your water right and spending a good deal of time, energy and money to make your drinking water safe.

The quality of your drinking water dictates how efficiently your body functions in the same way that the quality of the petrol you put in your car determines how smoothly your engine runs. The purer your drinking water, the easier it is for your body to use. The purity of drinking water has become a major concern for many people these days as tap water has been shown to fall well short of what one could reasonably say is safe (*see* Chapter 3).

The purity of your drinking water can be tested using a very simple device called a TDS (total dissolved solids) meter. This measures the amount of hidden solid matter in water. It is a small hand-held device with two metal probes at one end. It's really worth your while investing in one as it's very cheap, about €20, and can be used to test a range of waters such as well water, river water, tap water and bottled water. You can purchase a TDS meter online at www.tdsmeter.com, or you can get one from companies that supply equipment for science laboratories in schools and universities.

To test the water, simply place the metal probes in a sample of water and press a button on the meter, which will then display a reading in parts per million.

Pure water will give a reading of zero or close to zero, whereas tap water usually gives a reading of between 400 and 500 parts per million. Bottled waters show a lot of variation, between 150 and 500 parts per million. The best bottled waters, such as Spa mineral water from Belgium, has just under 150 parts per million. You are aiming for something between zero and 150, which represents relatively pure water containing less dissolved solid matter.

The level of purity of your water supply is important but even more important is the electronic structure of the water molecules, which is determined by the source of the water. If the source of the water is a county council treatment plant and the water has reached your home via metal or plastic pipes, it will have an undesirable structure. If it has come via a natural route – stream, river, well or melting glacier – it is likely to have a structure that is in harmony with your body and so be much more available to the cells of the body, or bioavailable.

For this reason, the best water on the planet is glacial water as it has been locked away within a glacier for thousands of years. These glaciers are found in Pakistan, Norway, Tibet and Chile. An example is Isklar from Norway. Very good water also comes from artesian wells, such as Spa mineral water from the town of Spa in Belgium, which has won numerous prizes.

If you wish to purify your water at home, get a distillation unit, which collects boiled water as steam and then condenses it back to a liquid. Store this water in glass bottles or earthenware containers. This water will be much purer and may be much more bioavailable.

Good Bacteria

You may be surprised that I list good bacteria as the second most important food. It is placed high up the list of important foods because it is critical for human health. As I mentioned in Chapter 4, 90 per cent of the cells that make up your body are actually bacteria, the very thing we have learned to be frightened of. Most bacteria are beneficial for human health and very, very few are harmful. Think of bacteria in a positive light as they are your first line of defence; put simply, you would not exist without them.

As mentioned in Chapter 4, all surfaces of the body have a thick coating of bacteria. These surfaces include the skin, the respiratory tract (nose to lungs), the digestive tract (all the way from the mouth to the anus), the urethra and the vagina. You cannot *see* these bacteria as they are microscopic in size and so can only be *seen* with the aid of a powerful microscope. Your body is home to no less than ninety trillion bacteria. We are basically a bacterial colony with only ten trillion human cells; hence, we are composed of many more bacterial cells than human cells – nine times more to be exact.

These bacteria are un*seen* and unsung heroes. They act as an interface between you and the environment in which you live. They exist to serve you in amazing ways.

They are your single most important defence against foreign microbes such as bad bacteria, viruses and other invaders. The gut bacteria in particular are an integral part of your immune system. These wonderful little bacteria supply you with a range of vitamins, including some B vitamins – vitamin B1, B2, B5 and B6 – and vitamin K, which is important in blood clotting. Recent research suggests that the gut flora may actually produce many more micronutrients than previously thought. The gut flora aids all aspects of gut function mainly by regulating the acid–alkaline balance in different parts of the gut. It also assists with bowel function; when the colonic flora goes out of balance, constipation or diarrhoea results.

The flora in the colon does something else that is quite amazing. It is able to digest some of the fibre in foods such as beans, lentils and legumes; it converts the fibre into short chain fatty acids (SCFAs), which have amazing beneficial consequences for you. These are acetic, propionic, butyric, lactic, hippuric and orotic acids. The most important of these acids is probably butyric acid, which forms the main food for the cells that line the colon. Without sufficient butyric acid, the lining of the colon becomes inflamed, and colitis, also called ulcerative colitis, begins. Colitis increases your risk of developing bowel cancer (*see* Chapter 4). A disturbance in the bacterial flora in the gut is now known to play a major role in the onset of colitis. As a consequence, most good gastroenterologists now prescribe probiotics for patients with this condition. Butyric acid is also known to be a key substance in the prevention of colonic cancer and possibly other cancers such as breast, prostate and liver cancer.

A number of these SCFAS, especially acetic and lactic acid, combine to produce an acidic environment that inhibits nasty pathogens such as typhoid bacteria. These SCFAS not only inhibit the growth of outside invaders but they also help to prevent the overgrowth of normal constituents of the gut flora, such as *Candida albicans*. So, when travelling to a foreign country, it is a good idea to take lots of good bacteria in the form of probiotic capsules to prevent traveller's diarrhoea. Also, if you are going to an area of the world where typhoid, cholera or dysentery may be present, it is really important to protect yourself with regular probiotic supplementation.

The benefits of these microscopic creatures are felt far beyond the gut. Propionic acid, for example, helps balance hormonal levels via its effects on the liver. Good bacteria have widespread positive effects on virtually all aspects of body function. They cooperate with you and live in harmony with you and ensure you remain healthy. To disturb the flora by using antibiotics unnecessarily or taking artificial sweeteners, both of which are known to disturb bacteria, is really a shame. One of the reasons why I wrote my first book *Alternatives to Antibiotics* was because I was shocked about the blatant over-prescription and abuse of antibiotics by doctors.

It is sad to *see* so few people, especially children, in the modern world using live bacterial foods. As we know, virtually all of the milk products used by people in Europe and North America are made from pasteurised milk. If, like most people, you don't have access to live cultures in milk products, use a probiotic supplement in the form of a capsule or powder, available from health shops. One of the best probiotic brands on the market is OptiBac as their product formulations have been well thought out and are based on sound medical research. Some commercial yoghurts have live cultures but unfortunately also have added sugar. It is best to avoid such yoghurts and don't give them to children, especially young children, as sugar is addictive. The best solution is to make your own yoghurt from raw milk, which is incredibly simple. Just take a look at one of the many demonstration videos on YouTube.

I cannot overstate the importance of the bacterial flora to human health. If you do nothing I suggest in this book other than take good bacteria every day, you will be doing yourself a huge favour.

Fats and Protein

After water and bacteria, the rest of your body is mainly made up of fats and proteins. Every cell in your body has a cell membrane around it that controls what enters and leaves the cell. The cell membrane is made up mostly of fat (phospholipid bilayer, to give it its technical name) with protein and cholesterol scattered throughout. You can *see* from Figure 6.2 that the cell membrane is composed of an outer layer of fat and an inner layer of fat; hence the term lipid bilayer. You can also *see* that this bilayer has proteins embedded in it. These proteins serve to regulate the transport of substances into and out of the cell, as well as transmitting messages to the cell. Cholesterol forms the third component of all cell membranes. So fat constitutes a major part of the cell membrane. This is why fat is so important in the diet.

Figure 6.2: *Components of a Cell Membrane*

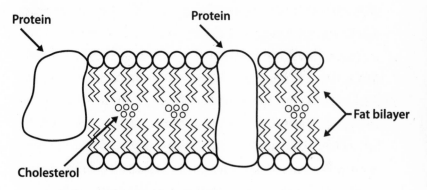

Two layers of fat (fat bilayer) are the basic component.
Protein and cholesterol are also components.

Source: McKenna, J.E., *Good Food: Can You Trust What You Are Eating?* Dublin: Gill & Macmillan, 2013: 44.

Inside the cell are many structures, such as the nucleus that contains DNA or genetic material and the mitochondrion that releases energy from food. Each of these structures has its own membrane, which is also mostly made up of fat and protein, as well as cholesterol.

A good analogy would be a house that is made up of exterior walls (the cell membrane) and interior walls that divide the house into rooms, each with its own function (the sub-cellular structures). However, while the exterior walls of a house may be made of bricks or blocks and the internal walls of a different material such as plasterboard, this is not true of the cell, in which all the membranes are made of the same materials – fat, protein and cholesterol.

When I was growing up, my mother and grandmother knew this, as did everyone else's. All cultures on this planet know that fat and protein (and cholesterol) are vital for survival. Some traditional tribal peoples such as the Inuit eat little else. They survive mostly on fat, combined with protein. Cholesterol is found in the same foods as animal fat.

Then along came Western scientists and decided they knew better. They decided to reduce the fat in our diet by demonising the most important type of fat, animal fat (saturated fat), such as that in butter, cheese, meat and so on. Science, the god of truth, issued words of warning that animal fats cause heart disease. Unfortunately, some foolish politicians in the USA listened to this message and even set up a Senate committee to investigate. The result was the greatest lie I have ever heard spoken. There is absolutely no evidence linking heart disease with dietary fat.

Because of public outcries by certain scientists and doctors back in the early 1980s and because of four large studies from different countries that effectively disproved the fat–heart disease link, in 1989 the US government asked the Surgeon General's Office to produce evidence linking animal fat in the diet with heart disease. They could not produce the evidence and it took no less than eleven years for them to state this; it was only in 1999, long after the message had been ingrained in everyone's brain, that they quashed the study, with no public admission that they could not find the evidence to support their promotion of a low-fat diet.

Fat and protein (and cholesterol) are the building blocks of your body. They are essential components of your cells. Cells are grouped together to form tissues with special functions, for example muscle tissue, and tissues are grouped together to form organs. So it's easy to *see* how important fats and protein are to your whole body. Fats and protein are critically important for a growing child, whose body is creating new cells all the time. However, they are critically important for adults as well as they are needed to repair and replace old cells.

Since all of the membranes in a cell are mostly made of fat, this constitutes the single most important food group to eat every day. Let's look at fats in a bit more detail.

Fats

The study of fats can *see*m quite confusing with the use of numerous terms such as saturated fat, monounsaturated fat, polyunsaturated fat, trans fat, and omega 3 and omega 6 fats, to name just a few. Very bamboozling! However, it doesn't need to be.

Saturated fats are found in animal fats for the most part and in some tropical oils such as coconut oil (I will use the terms saturated fat and animal fat interchangeably here). They tend to be solid or semi-solid at room temperature, e.g. butter. This solidity helps to add shape and structure to cell membranes, giving them the necessary stiffness and integrity. Therefore, most of the fat in a membrane is composed of saturated fat. The body regards saturated fats as essential and so goes to the trouble of making them if you do not eat enough in your diet. The body has a clever way of making them from carbohydrates. (The workings of the body and nature as a whole are simply amazing.) In my opinion, saturated or animal fat is the single most important part of a healthy diet, after water and bacteria of course. Here are my reasons for saying this:

- Saturated fats are vital for the structure and function of all cells.
- Saturated fats are important for the absorption of fat-soluble vitamins: A, D, E and K.
- Saturated fats protect against heart disease by lowering a substance in the bloodstream called Lp(a), which is an indicator of susceptibility to blocked arteries.
- Saturated fats protect your liver from toxins such as alcohol.
- Saturated fats boost the immune system.
- Some saturated fats have antimicrobial properties; they protect against harmful microbes in the gut.

Saturated fats are quite stable and so do not go rancid easily. They are useful in cooking and baking.

Unsaturated fats are divided up into **monounsaturated** and **polyunsaturated fats**. Monounsaturated fat is the most like saturated fat as it is chemically quite similar: it has only one double bond, while saturated fat has no double bonds. Your body can convert a saturated fat into a monounsaturated fat. A good example of a source of monounsaturated fat is olive oil, but it is also found in certain nuts, such as almonds, pecans, cashews and peanuts, and in avocados. Like saturated fats, monounsaturated fats are quite stable, do not go rancid easily and can be used in cooking.

Polyunsaturated fats have two or more double bonds and so are quite different from saturated fats. These cannot be made by the body and so they are called essential fats, since they must be obtained from the diet. The two poly-unsaturated fats found most commonly in our diet are linoleic acid (omega 6) and linolenic acid (omega 3). You have read about omega 6 and omega 3 already (*see* Chapters 3 and 5). Linoleic acid or omega 6 is found in many vegetable oils, such as sunflower, sesame and evening primrose oils; linolenic acid or omega 3 is found in fish oil and flax*seed* oil. Polyunsaturated fats or oils are quite different in that they are liquid at room temperature and go rancid very quickly, especially linolenic acid (omega 3). They should never be heated or used in cooking.

All fats found in nature are a combination of saturated and unsaturated fats. For example, olive oil is 75 per cent monounsaturated, 13 per cent saturated and 12 per cent polyunsaturated. Lard or pork fat is 48 per cent monounsaturated, 40 per cent saturated and 12 per cent polyunsaturated. The amount of omega 3 and omega 6 in animal fat varies with the diet of the animal.

All forms of fat are essential for good health. Lately, I have begun to ask my patients to increase the amount of animal fat in their diet to compensate for the misinformation being given by the health authorities.

Fats and proteins tend to occur together in nature. Milk, for example, is rich in protein but also has a full complement of fats. Eggs are probably the best and most complete food on the planet as they have a wonderful combination of fat and protein. Breast milk is yet another example. Fat and protein are buddies because they form the cell membranes of all living creatures. They are inseparable, or so it *seems*. Interestingly, the third component of cell membranes (cholesterol) is found in the same foods as fat and protein. So they are like the three musketeers.

Protein

After water, good bacteria and fat, protein forms the fourth most important part of a healthy diet. It is often written in school books and university textbooks that protein is the most important part of the diet, but this is simply not true. Proteins are also described as the building blocks of the body and this also is untrue. They do assist in the structure of membranes, muscle tissue and other tissues, but it is misleading to think of them as the sole building blocks. If we use the analogy of the walls of a house, the bricks would represent the fat bilayer and the mortar would represent the protein, but both are necessary to form a solid structure.

There are many types of protein, each playing a different role in the body: structural proteins, which form part of the cell membrane; enzymes, which speed up chemical reactions; hormones, which control chemical reactions and other body functions; and antibodies, which, as you may know, form part of the immune defence.

All proteins consist of a long chain of amino acids. There are twenty-two different amino acids and the body needs all twenty-two to build the huge array of proteins needed. Your body can actually manufacture some of these amino acids; it can in fact make fourteen of the twenty-two. The body cannot make the remaining eight amino acids and so these have to be obtained from the diet.

If the protein you consume as food contains all twenty-two amino acids, it is called a complete protein. Complete proteins are therefore the best form of protein to eat. They are found in foods from animal sources, such as meat, poultry, eggs, dairy produce, fish and shellfish.

If one or more of the twenty-two amino acids is missing, the protein is referred to as incomplete; plant proteins such as wheat are generally incomplete. So foods with incomplete protein would include grains, pulses, nuts and vegetables. However, by combining plant proteins, such as pulses and grains, it is possible to supply the body with a full complement of amino acids. This is why vegetarians have to mix their foods carefully so as not to be become protein deficient.

Primitive people around the world thrived for centuries on a diet composed mainly of protein and fat with occasional fruit, seeds and nuts. Many still thrive today on such a diet. Studies done on these people testify to their high level of health. The fat and protein is invariably animal in origin. However, there are people on a purely plant-based diet who also have a very high level of health. What nobody disagrees about is the very low level of health that people on a diet of mostly processed foods have. This is the worst diet for many reasons, not least its toxicity, which I have already looked at. However, there is also a genetic reason. Genetically we have greatest difficulty with cereals, processed milk and the array of chemicals added to foods.

We have survived mainly on animal produce for centuries, as many traditional tribal cultures still do. It is only more recently that farming entered the picture and humans became exposed to cereals such as wheat and rye, for example. As yet our DNA has not had time to adjust to accommodate these changes to our diet. Until this change happens, cereal allergies will top the list of food allergies experienced by humans.

What Are the Effects of a High Protein Diet?

There are many people who claim that too much protein in the diet is harmful. However, this simply does not fit the facts. Scientific evidence suggests that high levels of protein in the diet, especially animal protein, lead to longevity (Shils *et al.*, 1994). Russians from the Caucasus Mountains, who are famous in Europe for their health and longevity, eat a diet with lots of meat and dairy produce. This is one example of many. The claim that animal products shorten one's life span is not true. A high-protein diet is essential for good health.

A diet that is completely devoid of animal produce and that is based purely on plant produce can be problematic. A vegetarian diet often lacks sufficient vitamin D (and other fat-soluble vitamins), leading to poor absorption of minerals such as calcium. Also, phytates in grains block the uptake of a number of minerals in the gut; this is why it is essential to predigest cereals by fermenting or soaking them in water before using them in cooking. In the modern world this often does not happen. One common deficiency in animals fed on grains is zinc deficiency. This can often lead to physical deformities. In humans, zinc deficiency is not uncommon and can result in learning difficulties, mental retardation, delayed sexual maturation, slow growth and many other problems. Up to one-third of the world's population is at risk of zinc deficiency; that's how important a public health issue it is. It is also the fifth leading risk factor for disease in the developing world.

Simply put, the ideal form of protein in the diet is animal protein as this form of protein is complete and is easier for the gut to digest. I grew up listening to my family speak about the importance of protein; I also learned about it at school and later at university. Later still, in Africa, I saw the devastating effects of a lack of protein in the diet of young children, many of whom died as a result.

These days, there is a lot of nonsense being spoken and written about animal protein and animal fat. I can say without reservation that the basic foods needed every day in the diet are fat and protein, in that order.

Carbohydrates

Carbohydrates are described as the energy foods or fuel for your body. It is true that carbohydrates do indeed provide a source of energy in the form of glucose. All living creatures, plants and animals alike, use glucose as a source of energy. However, glucose is not the only source of energy. You may not know that fats are a much better source of energy in that they provide many more calories per gram. Carbohydrates include starchy foods, such as potato, rice, pasta and bread, as well as sugary foods, such as table sugar (sucrose), fruit sugar (fructose) and milk sugar (lactose).

Starchy foods such as potatoes are made up of long chains of glucose molecules. In the process of digestion, this long chain of glucose molecules gets broken down into individual glucose molecules, which are then transported across the gut wall and into the bloodstream. It is dangerous to have too much glucose in the bloodstream so the hormone insulin escorts it out of the bloodstream and into the cells of the body, where it is broken down to release energy. If a cell has sufficient supplies of stored energy, the glucose is stored for future use.

Although glucose is used in nature to provide energy, we do not actually need to ingest it. The body has a very clever way of making glucose from fat in a process called gluco-neogenesis. This is because there was little starch available in the primitive diet so the body needed other ways of getting a reliable supply of energy. Many people have survived without eating carbohydrates at all. Some still do. Examples include the Maasai, the Inuit, and the pre-Columbian Indians of North America.

It is really only in the last century that the Western diet has included so much refined sugar. Prior to this, the only sugar consumed was for the most part honey or fruit sugar. Where sugar and starch is found in nature, one also finds an array of vitamins and minerals, fibre, enzymes and also some fat and protein. So nature provides the enzymes to digest the carbohydrate as well as essential vitamins and minerals to assist with its absorption and metabolism. Nature also provides fibre to slow down the rate of absorption of glucose and also to assist with bowel evacuation.

The refining of carbohydrate strips the food of a lot of these extra vitamins, minerals, enzymes and fibre, making it harder for the body to digest and metabolise the food. This means that your body's reserves of vitamins and minerals get called upon, so depleting you of these essential elements. Because of the lack of fibre in refined carbohydrates, glucose levels in the bloodstream can rise sharply and ultimately predispose you to diabetes.

The introduction of refined carbohydrates to isolated communities invariably led to a whole string of health problems, appropriately called the diseases of civilisation – heart disease, diabetes, hypertension, obesity, arthritis and so on. Why is refined sugar in particular so damaging?

Table sugar or sucrose, to give it its chemical name, is made up of two sugars called glucose and fructose. You are probably quite familiar with these already as both are used in the home for baking and cooking. Glucose is relatively harmless as it is nature's energy-giving food and is used by every cell in every animal and plant. The real culprit is fructose; small quantities in fruit are fine, but in large quantities it wreaks havoc with the body's chemistry. It is described by some as a toxin or poison and I believe that is correct. It wreaks havoc with the liver's ability to function in much the same way that alcohol does; in fact, many of the complications associated with alcohol toxicity mimic the complications associated with fructose toxicity.

As mentioned above, all cells in the body can use glucose for energy or store it for future use. However, only the liver can use fructose, so the majority of the fructose absorbed goes straight to the liver and this is where all the damage is done. High amounts of fructose deplete the liver cells of energy, cause inflammation (hepatitis), and lead to the production of uric acid, which *see*ms to be a key substance in causing a chain of additional health problems. What is interesting about the metabolism of fructose in the liver is the fact that most of it is converted to fat. This increase in the production of fat leads to an increase in bad cholesterol (LDL), which is implicated in heart disease – hence the established link between sugar and heart disease. This increased production of fat also leads to increased fat in the liver (fatty liver) and other organs and the deposition of fat intra-abdominally (beer belly). Fructose does indeed appear to be the underlying cause of the obesity epidemic, as I have described in my book *The Big Fat Secret.*

As I have mentioned, in the mid-1970s US food manufacturers decided to use a substance called high fructose corn syrup (HFCS) to replace fat as it was very sweet and it was very cheap. The food chemists knew the consequences of using HFCS as the harmful effects of high levels of fructose were well documented in the 1950s and 1960s, and were highlighted in many of Professor John Yudkin's books (Yudkin was a professor of physiology in London who did a lot of research on fructose). However, they went ahead and did it anyhow, and soon HFCS found its way into almost every processed food and drink.

The truth is that carbohydrates are not essential unless you are doing a lot of physical work or are a professional athlete. If you do eat carbohydrates, eat only wholemeal foods. However, all wholegrains contain phytic acid, which, as mentioned, blocks the absorption of certain minerals such as calcium, magnesium, zinc and copper; they are also hard to digest because of enzyme inhibitors that interfere with the action of digestive enzymes in the gut. This is why, as mentioned above, it is good to either soak or ferment grains before using them. Many people who are allergic to cereals such as wheat may find that they can tolerate the cereal if it is predigested by soaking or by fermenting it. So, if you like to eat porridge oats, soak them overnight before cooking, as this will make them easier to digest. Avoid sugar and all foods containing it, and avoid any food containing

HFCS, which is labelled as corn syrup, or fructose syrup or glucose-fructose.

So, in summary, water, good bacteria and fats are the most important food groups, followed by protein. Carbohydrates are the least important food group and the least important **macro**nutrient (carbohydrate, protein and fat). They are even less important than the **micro**nutrients, minerals and vitamins, which I shall discuss next.

Minerals

Minerals, in my opinion, are the most interesting and exciting part of our diet. They illustrate very well the link between us and the planet we inhabit. They also reflect our true origins as stellar beings. They are more important than vitamins by far. Allow me to explain what I mean.

Plants make food that feeds the rest of creation. They do this by absorbing carbon dioxide (CO_2) from the air and water (H_2O) from the soil to make food in the form of glucose (which contains carbon, hydrogen and oxygen atoms). Plants also use nitrogen to make protein. Despite the fact that air contains lots of nitrogen, plants are not able to use atmospheric nitrogen and so they depend on a supply of nitrogen from the soil. However, they cannot use this inorganic nitrogen from soil and so they form a partnership with certain bacteria called nitrogen-fixing bacteria, which convert the nitrogen in soil into a form that plants can use called organic nitrogen. In return, the plant supplies the bacteria with food. Good trade! In this way plants are able to make protein.

Plants also absorb many minerals from soil. These minerals get passed to you directly when you eat the plant raw or indirectly via animals that eat the plants. The mineral content of the soil is the single most important factor in human nutrition. If the soil is deficient in minerals, then your body will be deficient. Testing soil for its mineral content is vitally important. So, if you grow your own vegetables, fruit or crops, get your soil tested regularly. If it is found to be deficient in one or more mineral, then correct the deficiency by adding a dressing of minerals and take a multi-mineral supplement yourself.

Minerals not only connect us to the very earth we stand on, they also connect us to the universe. In particular, they connect us to dying stars in the universe, from which all minerals – calcium, magnesium, phosphorus, zinc, iron and so on – originate. Hydrogen is the simplest atom. In stars like our sun, hydrogen atoms fuse together to form helium. To make more complicated atoms, you need much higher temperatures, which only exist when a star is dying. When this occurs, atoms such as carbon, oxygen and nitrogen (the basis of all food) can be formed and life can become possible. With even higher temperatures, other bigger atoms can be formed, such as iron, zinc and calcium. As a star dies, it explodes and scatters these atoms across the universe, allowing life to occur and you and me to exist. Without minerals, nothing else would exist. They are truly bits of magic.

We need seven minerals in large amounts – calcium, magnesium, phosphorus, potassium, sodium, chloride and sulphur – and many minerals in trace amounts, too many to list. The exact number of trace minerals essential for life probably equates to the number of minerals found in the earth's crust, which is quite a lot. The role of many of these trace minerals is not known. In other words, we have much to learn.

We get most of our minerals and trace minerals from water, raw food or lightly cooked food, and sea salt. Many of the African tribes I have visited actually add soil to food and to water, which is fascinating. In Europe many people use clay in food; for example, the French and people in Alpine regions, such as the Germans, Swiss, Austrians and Italians, add bentonite clay to food. Most of the minerals we need are found mostly in food. These minerals play vital roles in many of the chemical reactions that take place in our cells. For example, iron is a positively charged mineral that binds to negatively charged sites on the haemoglobin molecule in red blood cells. In the act of binding, the iron changes the shape of the haemoglobin molecule, opening up a space for oxygen to bind to haemoglobin. So, without iron, it would not be possible for oxygen to be transported around the body in the red blood cells. This oxygen is critical for cells to be able to convert food to energy.

Without iron, you would not exist as you would not be able to get the benefit of the food you eat. But all minerals play equally important roles. Even though some minerals are only need in tiny amounts, they are still essential for your survival. Interestingly, the body is aware that too much of any mineral can be toxic and so the gut only absorbs what it needs at any one time. So, we need a steady supply of minerals in our food on a daily basis to keep us 'topped up', so to speak.

There are a number of reasons why you may become deficient in minerals. Maybe the soil your vegetables are grown in is deficient; maybe the grass the animals in your food chain ate was deficient; maybe your gut is not functioning correctly; maybe other foods in your diet are blocking the absorption of these minerals.

As soil analyses have proved and tests done on fruits and vegetables have shown, the soil in market garden areas around many cities is depleted of minerals. Avoid supermarket vegetables and fruit, and rather *seek* out local farmers' markets or, better still, grow your own produce. Many people are now opting for the latter and there has been a huge surge in the 'grow your own' movement. Alternatively, make sure you and your loved ones take a multi-mineral supplement daily, especially if you are eating processed foods.

Selenium

The single most important mineral in relation to cancer risk is undoubtedly selenium. The reason for this is that there appears to be a strong association between selenium deficiency and cancer.

This has been demonstrated many times in animals. More recently, studies have shown that many cancer patients have low levels of selenium. In addition, cancer appears to be more common in areas where the soil is deficient in this important mineral. Also, cancer is more common in areas of the world where there is known to be a deficiency of selenium (National Research Council, 1989).

The importance of selenium relates to its antioxidant activity. It is essential for the function of an enzyme that protects every cell in the body from attack by viruses, chemicals, metals and other toxins. It works with vitamin E, another antioxidant, to protect the cell against dangerous carcinogens.

Good sources of selenium are fish, grains and Brazil nuts. This, of course, supposes that the grains and nuts have been grown in soil that has good levels of selenium.

Farmers are usually not bothered if their soil is deficient in selenium as it is not an essential mineral for plants and so does not affect their health.

In 1984, the Food and Nutrition Board in the USA reviewed the literature on selenium and cancer and stated that 'Low selenium intakes or decreased selenium concentrations in the blood are associated with increased risk of cancer in humans' (National Research Council, 1989: 10). It also found that the anti-cancer effect of selenium *see*ms to be more common in males than in females and is more protective against colon cancer and lung cancer (National Research Council, 1989).

Supplementation of the diet or drinking water with selenium appears to offer significant protection against a range of cancers, at least in laboratory animals. Selenium has also been shown to protect against a range of carcinogens, including certain metals (National Research Council, 1989). In fact, one of the ways of counteracting the negative effects of metals in the body is to use antioxidants such as selenium and vitamin E.

I test my patients for mineral deficiencies, and selenium deficiency is not uncommon.

I usually advise taking a broad vitamin and mineral supplement, which contains good levels of selenium and vitamin E, for a period of time and then retesting. However, it is possible to take selenium alone; if you wish to do this, use a dosage of 200 micrograms daily with food. Do not exceed this dosage as toxicity may result. Take vitamin E simultaneously as selenium needs vitamin E to function effectively.

Vitamins

Many people regard vitamins and minerals as somewhat similar. However, there are some key differences. First, vitamins are complex molecules composed of carbon, hydrogen, oxygen and nitrogen, whereas minerals are very basic structures and usually exist as a charged atom (ion) or as a salt. Second, because of their chemical complexity, vitamins are easily damaged by factors such as temperature, pressure and radiation; minerals are not damaged by these factors. Therefore, the freshness of food affects vitamin content but not mineral content. If a mineral is present in a food it will remain until the food is eaten. However, cooking methods can alter the vitamin content significantly; for example, vitamin C is largely destroyed by cooking. All minerals must be obtained from food, whereas some vitamins, such as vitamin D, can be manufactured by the body.

Many vitamins need additional co-factors to operate effectively. For example, vitamin C needs certain minerals, rutin, bioflavonoids and other substances to function. Vitamins often do not exist as single entities but as a group of complex molecules, many of which have yet to be discovered. Vitamin B complex has at least seventeen components that we know of, which appear to work together synergistically. Vitamin D has twelve components and vitamin P at least five. Because of their complex nature and their many constituents, vitamins are very difficult to manufacture in pill form, making food (not supplements) the best means of obtaining them.

For the most part, vitamins *seem* to work as antioxidants, which protect the cells from damage, or as facilitators of enzyme reactions, i.e. they work as co-factors helping certain chemical reactions to take place. Vitamin C is an antioxidant, while vitamin B1 is a co-factor.

The food processing industry may add vitamins at low levels to foods for advertising purposes, but then proceed to damage these vitamins by subjecting them to high heat and pressure. In addition, sugar, which is added to most processed foods, depletes the body of some of the B vitamins. Long periods of high heat used in canning foods can also destroy certain vitamins. Interestingly, sun drying can actually enhance vitamin content, for example sun-dried fruits. The traditional methods of treating foods were much wiser and safer.

Vitamin A

Vitamin A is particularly worthy of mention. It is the reason why I got interested in nutrition. I remember reading an article on the positive effects of vitamin A supplementation in reducing infections in children born to mothers who were HIV positive. It was a study carried out in Durban, South Africa in the early 1990s. It made me acutely aware of why HIV infection is so prevalent in southern Africa: it all comes down to poor nutrition.

Because I have always had a strong interest in digestive problems, vitamin A is of interest to me as it assists in the digestion of protein in the stomach by stimulating the secretion of digestive juices. However, it does a lot more than this. According to nutrition expert Dr Weston Price, the body cannot utilise protein, minerals or water soluble vitamins (C and B complex) without sufficient vitamin A. Hence, vitamin A could be regarded as the single most important vitamin and possibly one of the most important micronutrients. Vitamin A from animal sources – eggs, liver, cod liver oil, seafood, milk, butter – is much easier for the body to use since it is in the form of retinol, the form the body needs; vitamin A from vegetable sources – any green, yellow or orange vegetables such as spinach, cabbage, peppers and carrots – is harder for the body to use as the vegetable form of vitamin A, beta carotene, needs to be converted to retinol in the body. The conversion of beta carotene to retinol can be difficult for some people, especially infants and young children, diabetics and those with an under-active thyroid (hypothyroidism). According to Dr Price's findings, and to the findings of many other researchers since, the healthiest people on the planet have the highest intake of vitamin A.

Vitamin A is probably the most powerful antioxidant of all. It has been researched extensively for its ability to prevent cancer, even in those at greater risk than the average person. The increase in incidence of certain types of cancer has been linked by some researchers to low vitamin A levels (Boik, 2001). The results of these studies show that lung cancer in particular is associated with low levels of vitamin A in the diet, as well as cancers of the larynx, mouth, oesophagus, stomach, colon, prostate and cervix (Boik, 2001). Recent research from Japan has shown that those who consume foods rich in vitamin A are less likely to develop a whole range of cancers (Tsubono *et al.*, 1999). Research from the Philippines has shown that the administration of vitamin A has the ability to reduce cellular abnormalities (a pre-cancer state), especially in the mouth and the cervix (De Luca, 1995).

Vitamin A deficiency is one of the most common and most serious nutritional deficiencies across the globe. Severe vitamin A deficiency occurs commonly in the third world and in my work in Africa I have *seen* lots of children with it. Interestingly, I have also *seen* evidence of it here in Europe among people with malabsorption and people using slimming pills, which block the absorption of fat in the gut, causing fatty stools. Signs of vitamin A deficiency include:

- Dry eyes
- Difficulty *see*ing well in dim light (night blindness)
- Dry skin
- Recurrent infections
- In children in Africa, poor growth and development (failure to thrive)

Vitamin A is one of the fat-soluble vitamins and is stored in the body, so it is possible to overdose on it. The recommended intake of retinol for adults is approximately 1000 micrograms a day. Pregnant women and breast-feeding mothers require a little bit more, up to 1200 micrograms a day. It is possible to use higher doses, but remember that it can be toxic at very high doses. It is best to eat lots of foods rich in vitamin A, which is what nature intended, rather than take pills.

Enzymes

If I had written this book twenty years ago, I probably would not have included a section on enzymes. The study of enzymes and the role they play in nature is relatively new in the field of nutrition. Today, we have identified many thousands of enzymes that *seem* to play a role in just about every chemical reaction that happens in the body. They basically speed up chemical reactions by bringing all the necessary components together to allow the reactions to happen. The enzymes employ minerals and vitamins to assist them in this.

When a vitamin or a mineral attaches to an enzyme to assist it in speeding up a chemical reaction, the vitamin or mineral is referred to as a co-factor. This is the principal role of vitamins and minerals. Zinc, for example, is known to be a co-factor in over 200 enzyme reactions in various parts of the body. When glucose enters the cell, it is broken down into carbon dioxide and water in a series of enzyme reactions. Magnesium and the B vitamins play roles as co-factors in some of these reactions.

The digestive enzymes in your digestive tract are one class of enzyme; these break down your food to facilitate its absorption across the gut wall. There are two other classes of enzyme as well. These are the metabolic enzymes, which facilitate all the chemical reactions in the cells of the body, and the food enzymes, which I will discuss now.

Raw food sometimes contains enzymes that help the process of digestion. In essence, the food is giving you a gift of digestive enzymes to ease the burden on your pancreas by making the job of converting the food into a bio-available form that much easier. Hence, raw food is an important part of any diet. We tend to eat raw fruit and sometimes raw vegetables in salads, and some people drink raw milk. People in more traditional, tribal cultures often eat some of their meat raw and on occasion their fish as well. What they do not eat raw or cooked, they ferment over a period of time, which can enhance the nutritional value of the food. Fermented dairy products, such as soured milk, are not only rich in bacteria but rich in enzymes as well. Fermented products such as fermented vegetables (sauerkraut) and fermented soya beans (tofu and miso) are really important to consume for this reason.

Grains, nuts and seeds are rich in enzymes but also contain enzyme inhibitors, so making them a bit hard on the digestive tract. To get rid of these enzyme inhibitors, certain techniques have been used over the centuries – sprouting, soaking the food in water with a little lemon juice added, fermenting, sourdough leavening. Most fruit and vegetables have little in the way of enzymes, with a few notable exceptions. Pineapple and pawpaw (papaya) are rich in enzymes and so are used by companies that manufacture digestive enzymes for sale in health shops. Many tropical fruits have enzymes, such as kiwis, avocados, mangoes, dates, bananas and plantains.

High heat destroys all the natural enzymes in food. The purpose of pasteurising milk is to kill bad bacteria by the use of high heat. This destroys not only all the bacteria but all the enzymes as well, so making the milk much harder to digest. The activity of one particular enzyme, called alkaline phosphatase, is measured after heating the milk; if it is zero then the milk can be deemed pasteurised.

It follows that cooking also destroys enzymes. You can see why people hold up a raw food diet as healthy. I am personally not a great fan of a raw food diet. I was brought up mostly on cooked foods and I have continued this pattern of eating. Mentally I understand the need for a lot of raw or fermented food in the diet, but emotionally I have not succumbed to the idea. I do eat salads (occasionally) and I do eat lot of fruit and try to source raw milk, but I am afraid to say the rest of my food is cooked. Ireland for me is too cold to survive on mostly raw or fermented foods. I hear others speak about nutrition and say that 80 per cent of your diet should be raw food. Good for them if they can do it, but personally I enjoy what I eat and have evolved a way of eating that is good for me. I am tuned in to my body well enough to know what it needs.

Salt

We humans evolved from the sea and the composition of our bodies reflects this.

I mentioned earlier in this chapter that we are mostly water. That water is mostly salted water: the water in our bloodstream and our tissue fluid contains dissolved sodium chloride. Both sodium and chloride are important for health.

Salt sold in supermarkets, like much of the food sold there, is highly refined. Even a lot of sea salt is refined as well. It undergoes chemical changes in the refining process, which removes most of the magnesium and other minerals. The best salt is sundried sea salt, which is not refined and so is rich not only in sodium chloride but in many other minerals as well. So it is best to buy salt in a health food shop and ask for unrefined, sundried sea salt or salt from the Himalayas.

SUMMARY

The main constituents of a healthy diet are water, good bacteria, fats, protein, minerals and vitamins, with a minimum amount of carbohydrate, unless you are expending a lot of energy at work. Part of the diet should be raw food.

The human body is very simple in one sense and highly complex in another. It needs basic, simple, natural foods, such as those mentioned in this chapter, to function effectively. The way these foods combine in the body to our benefit is truly magical and complex. We need to trust in nature and in the foods she provides us with.

We have been deliberately led away from this simple natural diet in favour of denatured food. We have been deliberately misled about cholesterol, about sugar and even about animal protein. If you confuse people enough, you can control them.

We have been poisoned with high fructose corn syrup, which causes severe health problems. Later in this book I will discuss aspartame, an artificial sweetener that is being blamed for the sudden rise in brain tumours since its introduction in 1981. We have been deliberately misinformed by governments, by the WHO, by the medical profession, by dieticians and by many other organisations and professional bodies. Why? For profit it would *see*m, via control of the food chain.

Let's now look at the elements of a healthy diet again from a different perspective, starting with water.

WATER

I grew up drinking well water and later tap water. At the age of fifteen, I went on a school trip to France and was surprised to *see* people drinking water from a plastic bottle. In my innocence I believed that water was free, plentiful and healthy to drink.

It is now almost impossible to find clean safe water to drink. We have polluted the water table and streams and rivers with agricultural chemicals. Tap water is laden with chemicals and because of the high solid content is unhealthy to drink. That leaves bottled water as the best option, even if it is in a plastic bottle. Alternatively, get a reverse osmosis filter to purify your tap water.

Spa mineral water is an excellent mineral water available in the UK but not in Ireland. It has a very low TDS level and so has a high level of purity. Artesian well water such as Spa, volcanic water such as Volvic and glacial water such as Isklar from Norway are good as they come from the belly of the earth or from melting glaciers. These are the purest forms of water.

There have been problems with bad bugs in the water supply to the tap in many counties. This can lead to acute illness. What is a bit more serious is the presence of metals in the water supply. A newspaper report from 2013 claimed that at least 30,000 households in Ireland could be at risk of lead poisoning from drinking water. Lead is a highly toxic metal, which is why it was removed from petrol, paint and solder. It causes chronic ill health.

Chlorine is added to tap water. Chlorine not only kills bad bacteria but it also kills the good bacteria in your body. Fluoride is also added to tap water. Fluoride is an enzyme inhibitor that can cause bone loss and has now been implicated in the development of bone cancer. This is good reason to ban the fluoridation of water. In 1990, the American National Toxicology Program reported a clear linkage between fluoridation and the malignant bone cancer osteosarcoma. This cancer is on the increase. It is almost invariably fatal and affects young children and adolescents (Epstein, 1998).

Avoid tap water, regardless of where you live, and try to get the best bottled water you can. The rationale behind water purification plants operated by your local council is to remove as much debris as possible and to kill bugs. In other words, the sole rationale is safety. It has nothing at all to do with producing water as close to the natural state as possible; it has nothing to do with producing healthy water for the human body. Safe water is not healthy water. The two objectives are poles apart. Chlorine will make your water safe, but who wants to drink swimming-pool water?

FATS

Animal fats and cholesterol have been demonised as striking people down in the prime of their lives. Doctors advise their patients to cut down on eggs, butter and cheese, and to eat lean meats. Everyone follows the same advice as they wish to prevent heart attacks. The advice is totally incorrect. First, the terminology is all wrong. Cholesterol and animal fat are completely different substances with completely different functions in the body. Cholesterol is not a fat at all. Chemically it bears no relation to fat. Second, the term 'bad cholesterol' is misleading, as all cholesterol is good and necessary. We should use the term LDL (low density lipo-protein) instead (LDL is the protein that carries cholesterol around the body). There is no need to add the word cholesterol after it.

Third, as stated earlier in this chapter, there is no hard scientific evidence to substantiate the idea that any type of fat is bad for you, including animal fat, and definitely no evidence that animal fat causes heart disease. The most famous medical study ever done on heart disease, the Framington Heart Study, has shown that there is no link with animal fat. So, why persist with this nonsense? You are being misled and misinformed and wrongly advised.

As I have shown in my book *The Big Fat Secret* (2012) there is definite hard scientific evidence linking sugar intake with heart disease. This information is kept hidden from you by lies, deceit and misinformation. However, it will not remain hidden for much longer.

So the controversy about fat and cholesterol is really just a smoke screen to hide the truth.

PROTEIN

There is much controversy surrounding the link between dairy products and cancer.

The link between the milk protein, casein, and various forms of cancer has been known for some time but was highlighted in 2006 with the publication of a book called *The China Study* by Dr Colin Campbell. In this book his research does indeed show a link between milk protein, casein, and the promotion of certain cancers, notably liver cancer. On the basis of this research it is possible to advise people to be cautious about commercial, pasteurised milk. However, there is no problem with the whey protein found in milk.

What I do not like about Campbell's book is his conclusion that not just dairy but all animal protein should be avoided. He spends most of the book advocating a vegan diet rather than dealing with the evidence from his research in China. For such an intelligent man he has some very fundamental errors in his conclusions. He ignores the many tribes of people in the world who have thrived on animal protein for centuries and who show no evidence of liver cancer or any other cancer. Some of these tribes, such as the Fulani and Maasai in Africa, consume a lot of milk protein. He ignores the fact that his source of casein was pasteurised milk, not raw milk. He does not consider that maybe it is the pasteurisation process that is altering the casein, making it promote cancer.

Until this controversy about casein is settled, I would advise caution in the use of pasteurised milk and would opt for raw milk. Avoid all commercial dairy products such as cheese, yoghurt and ice cream; cream and butter are composed of animal fat so should be okay to use. Better still, use goat's milk or sheep's milk, or an alternative. Very commercial products such as cow's milk are big business. Just because it is endorsed by your government or your health authority does not mean it is safe. My motto is: if there is the slightest risk of harm, avoid it completely.

FOOD ADDITIVES

You will learn quite soon via the national press about the damage that certain food additives are doing to our health. In particular there has been much research focused on the artificial sweeteners – aspartame, sucralose and acesulfame K. These sweeteners have been endorsed as safe yet they have consistently shown to be harmful to people and to experimental animals. They are found in many drinks, foods, conventional cold and flu medicines and even children's vitamin supplements (it is best to buy vitamin supplements in a health shop). Sucralose has been shown to damage the bacterial flora of the gut and predispose to colitis, Crohn's disease and bowel cancer. Aspartame has been shown to cause leukaemia in humans. So throw out the diet drinks and check all medicine for these additives.

Chapter 7
Where to Shop for Food

It is very easy to advise people on what to avoid in their diet, such as sugar, but much harder to advise them on where they can find suitable alternatives. It is also easy to tell people to avoid the supermarkets and buy from local markets, but for a number of reasons that may simply be impractical. It is also good advice to suggest that you should grow your own vegetables and potatoes, but again that simply may not be possible. In essence, you have to be pragmatic and do what you can to minimise your exposure to carcinogens in food and in the environment. All any of us can do is the best we can.

In this chapter I want to look at the pros and cons of visiting the supermarket and to give you some useful options if you decide to shop elsewhere. The objective is to take the process of buying food to a more conscious, more aware level. Trying to break old habits and choosing foods that you feel will strengthen your immunity is the key.

The real difficulty comes when you realise that the staple foods, such as regular tea and coffee, wheat bread and cow's milk, have to be reduced or avoided completely. That is a huge shift to make, but it is really important to know that life will not cease and there are good alternatives available. It is only by searching for these alternatives that you will find them. This can be a bit of a challenge, but it is well worth it. It will change your life in a very positive way.

Supermarkets control about 80 per cent of the grocery trade in the British Isles, and therefore, in essence, they control to a great extent what we eat. As you have learned in this book, certain foods switch on cancer genes and other foods switch on protective genes; so, by controlling what we eat, the supermarkets are effectively controlling our level of health. That's why it becomes so very important to change your ideas about what you buy and where you buy it.

It can be helpful to start viewing the supermarket as a health centre that sells you medicines that make you stronger. If you have a cold or flu, they sell lemons or vitamin C, and if you have cancer they sell you green tea, soya milk, certain spices, fruit, berries, vegetables and mushrooms. When you hold that mindset for a while you will start to view processed foods, such as pasteurised milk, pizza and ordinary wheat breads, as unhealthy and promoters of cancer. In other words, you will be scared to eat these processed foods in the same way that you would be scared to take medicine that was potentially harmful to you.

Look for organic meat, and organically and locally grown vegetables, fruit and cereals that have not been sprayed with chemicals and are not genetically modified; seek out gluten-free options, such as gluten-free oats. The use of local produce helps everyone in that it is more likely to be fresh and the cost of transporting it is lower.

Remember, when visiting a supermarket you are the one in control. If you can't find what you need, ask a manager. Supermarkets are very sensitive to the demands of their shoppers. Not enough of us challenge the supermarkets on the type of food they stock their shelves with – mostly unhealthy processed food. The truth about supermarkets is that at present they provide food that suits them first and foremost. They like food that has a long shelf life and can be transported with minimal spoilage. They also prefer large-scale production to ensure continuity of supplies and maximum profit. You have the power to change all of that.

When you do your weekly shopping, you're involved in the single most important act regarding the health not just of your family but of the nation as a whole. By selecting healthier options, such as lots of organic produce, and refusing to buy processed food, you are changing the face of Western civilisation. Your actions will support the decline of the companies that manufacture processed foods such as Kellogg's and Coca-Cola. By demanding organic chemical-free meat, fruit and vegetables, you will reduce the power of the chemical companies. If enough people do this, then perhaps farmers will be left to grow safe crops in the traditional manner, and the soil and the water table will no longer be polluted. By refusing to buy processed food, you are also decreasing the power that food companies have over politicians and the medical profession, as well as over advisory bodies to governments and international bodies such as the WHO.

You can now *see* that the simple act of shopping can have enormous consequences for the whole society. So, how do you break the supermarket habit? Well, it's a simple matter of changing your mindset before entering the shop. Focus your mind on foods that will boost the health of you and your loved ones; do not be conned by tempting deals. In other words, put your health before money. Focus your mind on rebuilding your body, not satisfying cravings. This requires self-discipline. Focus your mind on boundless energy, not tiredness and lethargy. When making your shopping list, include each of the following:

- Safe water
- Good bacteria
- Fats and oils
- Protein
- Minerals
- Vitamins
- Starch
- A few treats

In terms of safe water, try to buy your water in a glass bottle, such as San Pellegrino or Acqua Panna, or, if you can't find these, use Spa or Volvic.

To get good bacteria, the best option is to buy a yoghurt maker and make live yoghurt at home. Yoghurt makers are available on the internet (for example at www.lakeland. co.uk) or in any shop that sells kitchenware. If you don't have the time to make your own yoghurt or don't want to, then buy plain natural yoghurt (preferably not made from cow's milk) that has no added sugar and also buy a probiotic supplement in the health shop. Open the probiotic capsule, add a little of the contents to the yoghurt and leave at 37 degrees Celsius overnight. In the morning, take the yoghurt on an empty stomach and give the bacteria time (about thirty minutes) to multiply in the gut before eating breakfast. There are a few good live yoghurts available in some supermarkets, but they are best bought in health shops, farm shops or farmers' markets where you can be sure you're getting the real deal.

Fats and oils would include some of the following: fat for frying foods, fat for baking, olive oil for cooking and foods that contain healthy fats. When frying meat, for example, use lard or butter, as they are more stable at high temperatures. The best fat for baking is unquestionably lard; traditionally lard was the fat used in baking and some people are now reverting to it. Use virgin olive oil when cooking on low to medium heat, but try to avoid all other vegetable oils such as sunflower, sesame and corn oil. Buy foods that are rich in essential oils. For example, buy lots of free range eggs (duck or hen's), and organic beef and pork. Because many people are deficient in omega 3 oils, buy flaxseed – ground flaxseed such as Virginia Harvest is easiest to use – or buy fish oil and/or lots of oily fish.

As mentioned in Chapter 6, the best protein is animal protein as it has all twenty-two amino acids. Eat lots of organic lamb's liver when it's available, as well as other organic meats such as kidney and heart. Also, eat free range chicken and organic beef and pork. The best protein and the one that's easiest to digest is fish protein, but try to get fresh wild fish caught out at sea rather than the farmed variety. If you don't like eating meat, use lots of vegetable protein, especially soya. Make sure to combine vegetable proteins so that you get the full complement of amino acids.

As mentioned in Chapter 6, minerals come from the soil and if the soil has good levels of all minerals then vegetables grown in it and animals fed on it will supply your body with everything it needs. You can't really tell the mineral content of supermarket foodstuffs so just opt for organic. Learn which foods are rich in certain minerals. Everyone has the belief that dairy is the richest source of calcium but that's not the case. The food with the highest level of calcium is kelp. Also, goat's milk has more calcium than cow's milk. A great way to get your minerals is to drink fresh juice made from organic fruit and vegetables. Buy a good juicer and a book on how to make nourishing juices.

Buy lots of ingredients to make salads and have this raw food at least once a day.

When making a dressing for the salad, opt for olive oil and lemon juice. Use lemon in your tea as well and in carbonated water such as San Pellegrino. Every morning, start the day with a glass of lukewarm water with the juice of one lemon added to it.

Cereals can be a problem for our health for a variety of reasons, as I mention earlier in this book. Suffice it to say that if you want to eat cereals, try to buy organically grown cereals and pre-digest them, such as by soaking overnight. If you are Celtic in origin and have digestive problems, it may be wiser to avoid all cereals or to use them infrequently.

The best source of B vitamins is yeast, for example brewer's yeast, so favour foods that have yeast in them as it will boost your energy levels. Red wine is a good source of yeast, and it also contains the chemical resveratrol, which has anti-cancer properties. Other vitamins will come from animal fat – the fat-soluble vitamins are A, D and E – and from fruit and vegetables. Make sure to top up with vitamin C during the winter months, as fruit is scarce at this time of year and it is when people are most prone to colds and flu.

There is no harm in having an occasional treat. I have a weakness for apple pie and feel the need to treat myself every so often. It's not what you eat infrequently that matters, but rather what you eat daily. If you have an addiction to a particular food then you will have to avoid it; otherwise, enjoy the odd treat, especially if it raises your spirits.

GUIDELINES FOR GROCERY SHOPPING

1. No Children
When grocery shopping, it is best to leave the children at home with a relative or go shopping when they are in crèche. In this way you'll be better able to maintain your focus on buying healthy foods.

2. Use a Basket or Small Trolley
By using only a basket or a small trolley, you will be better able to limit your shopping to essentials. Alternatively, shop online. That way you can focus on the essentials and you don't have the extra burden of finding someone to look after the children.

3. Be Very Focused
Don't get distracted by special offers, good deals and other marketing ploys. Know what you want before you enter and wear blinkers until you find what you're looking for, then leave.

4. Ask a Lot of Questions
For example, ask supermarket staff how fresh the fruit and vegetables are, ask where the meats have come from, and take the names and addresses of the farmers who supplied these foods. It is best to speak with a manager only.

FARMERS' MARKETS AND FARM SHOPS

There is a gradually expanding interest in farmers' markets in Ireland and the UK. The number of farmers' markets is growing rapidly. The first farmers' market in the UK opened in 1997 in the west country and today there are approximately five hundred. In Ireland, there are almost ten operating in Dublin and around the Dublin area; in addition, many towns have a market once a week. Almost one-third of the population prefer to buy produce directly from the farmer because of the lack of middle men and because they can ask questions and get straight answers (Harvey, 2008). The human interaction in the process of buying what are critically important items for your well-being is very important; you are much more likely to buy from someone with whom you have had a positive inter-action and who you believe to be honest and trustworthy. People are fed up with being conned by adverts, posters, sponsorship of events and so on. Also, a farmer who sells directly to neighbours, friends, and the local community is much more likely to take greater care over the production of his food than a farmer who sells produce to a food manufacturer or to a meat factory.

The nice thing about farmers' markets is that there are two simple rules governing them. First, the food has to be produced locally, normally within a certain radius of the market. Second, the seller must be familiar with the production process so that they are able to field all manner of questions. Some people find these markets a bit more expensive than the local supermarket, which is true, but the reason for shopping here is the quality of the produce, which is well worth the extra cost, and ultimately it is about investing in your health and avoiding illness, which can be very costly.

By supporting your local farmers' market, you are supporting a revolution in the way food is produced and sold. You are supporting good farming practices, old traditional methods of farming and reconnecting people with the farmers. This interface between eater and producer is of profound importance, not just because you get better and safer produce, but because you are helping to protect our planet against any further damage by industrial farming methods.

Farm shops located on the farms themselves are an even better idea as you are more likely to *see* the animals face to face, so to speak, and you can inspect the fields in which the produce is grown. You can tell a lot about what happens on the farm by inspecting the livestock. For example, are the hens or ducks allowed to wander freely around the fields and are the cattle alert, but quiet? Also, are there flowers and herbs growing in the fields? Natural pastures will have different types of grasses, herbs and flowers in the same field.

The farmer in this instance is hardly likely to attract customers if his/her farm is run badly, so the presence of a farm shop is automatically a good sign. If someone in the shop is willing to show you around the farm, then or at some future time, this is also a very good sign. However, not all the produce in a farm shop may come from the one farm. Neighbouring farmers may sell their produce through this one outlet. But if the farms are nearby, it is relatively easy to cast an eye over these as well. Life-long relationships are made by buying your produce directly from the farmer, because if you are happy with the produce you will not want to buy from anywhere else. You will be able to eat wholesome, natural foods as I was lucky enough to do when I was a child.

Box schemes are yet another way of getting good produce if you do not wish to visit a local farmers' market or farm shop. Where I live there is a local producer of organically grown vegetables who supplies a range of vegetables delivered in a box to my home. This is an excellent way of getting deliveries of fruit and vegetables.

The other main way of accessing good produce is to use the internet. Search for 'organic produce' or 'organic farmers' and you will find a host of really useful information. Useful Irish websites are:

- www.irishfarmersmarkets.ie
- www.iofga.ie (Irish Organic Farmers' and Growers' Organisation)

These websites have their equivalents in other countries, such as www.farmersmarkets.net, www.farmshops.org.uk and www.alotoforganics.co.uk in the UK.

The Irish Organic Farmers' and Growers' Association has a directory of members and can put you in touch with a farmer or grower close to where you live. Their contact details are:

Unit 16A, Inish Carrig, Golden Island, Athlone, Co. Westmeath

Email: info@iofga.ie

Tel: 090 643 3680

If you give yourself time, you may be able to wean yourself away from the supermarket entirely. It is a matter of taking time to source alternative suppliers of basic food items, making sure the produce from these outlets is of good quality, and making sure that the price is right for you. It is good to shop in the same place to give people time to get to know you and what your tastes are. Prices can be negotiable, but wait for the people in the farm shop or at the stalls at the farmers' market to realise that you are a regular customer and they may be more flexible on price.

SUMMARY

The most important daily act you carry out is to buy food. Your choice of foods has enormous consequences for everyone. It determines to a great extent your level of health and that of your family. Deleting sugary foods from your shopping list has enormous political consequences, as Western civilisation to a large extent depends on the huge profits made by food companies. The 2012 London Olympics was sponsored by many of these companies.

Avoid the supermarket, except for a few essentials such as bottled water, fruit and vegetables. Try to purchase as much farm produce – meats, eggs and vegetables – as possible from farmers' markets or directly from the farmer. Try to use organic produce when available. If you wish to use milk, use only raw milk products.

Chapter 8
The Role of Stress in Cancer

D r Bernie Siegel is a retired surgeon from the USA who is famous for his work on the relationship between the patient and the healing process, on which he has written a number of books, including *Love, Medicine and Miracles*. Siegel has stated that almost everyone diagnosed with cancer had been through a very stressful period preceding the onset of the disease. I have found the same pattern in my practice. It *see*ms that stress is the straw that breaks the camel's back, so to speak.

Stress appears to have a weakening effect on the immune system in particular. If your immune system is healthy, it *see*ms that you are better able to deal with carcinogens that enter the body via water, food or other means. But if you experience a period of ongoing stress, your immune system is gradually weakened.

Case History – Frank: Colon Cancer
Frank had suffered from constipation for most of his life and then at the age of fifty was diagnosed with colon cancer. He was combining what natural and conventional medicine had to offer in an attempt to treat the cancer. I was guiding him about the best forms of treatment available in natural

medicine. One day he came to see me because he was very upset at something that had happened at home: he had been very angry at something his young son had done and had beaten him. This was something he had never done before and he was distraught. Frank was aware that he could die from cancer and lived with this reality. He loved his family and had become much closer to them since his diagnosis. This sudden venting of anger alarmed him and so he came to me for help.

I spent some time exploring Frank's history, especially his childhood, and learned that he was carrying a lot of anger against the Christian Brothers who had taught him at school. He had been beaten almost daily at school because he was dyslexic. He was also beaten at home on occasion by his father, but he felt that most of these beatings had some justification compared to the ones at school, which had none.

He had buried these feelings for years and it was only when he was faced with cancer that he sought help; he became more open to healing all aspects of himself, including his emotional stress. I explained to him that when you open yourself to healing, emotions from the past that had been buried can surface out of the blue and must be released. However, they must be released in a constructive way. Hurting his son had a very negative effect on Frank, as well as on his son. I asked him to apologise to his son and be open with him about what had happened.

I referred Frank to a colleague who is a psychiatrist. Instead of prescribing drugs for emotional stress, the psychiatrist asked Frank to use breathing techniques and visualisation to help reduce his stress levels. Frank gained great benefit from this treatment.

Frank's story is an example of how internal stressors, in this case anger and resentment, can disturb one emotionally. These kinds of stressors work at a subconscious level and constantly keep the nervous system on high alert. The body will release cortisol and adrenalin on an ongoing basis as a consequence. The effect of this is suppression of the immune system, making cancer more likely.

During the 1920s, Professor Hans Selye of the University of Prague carried out research on the negative effects of stress on the body (Selye, 1976). His years of medical research led him to propose a model (*see* Figure 8.1) to explain how stress affects us.

Figure 8.1: The Effects of Stress on the Body

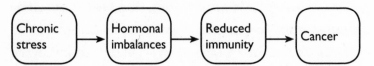

Source: Selye, H., *Stress in Health and Disease*, London: Butterworths, 1976.

Professor Selye proposed that chronic stress leads to the release of high levels of hormones from the adrenal glands – adrenalin and cortisol. The effects of cortisol, a steroid hormone, are to suppress immunity and the effects of adrenalin are to stimulate inflammation. As outlined earlier, both suppression of the immune system and inflammation favour the development of cancer.

Dr O. Carl Simonton, who was famous for his pioneering work with cancer patients, noted that that a high percentage of his patients had experienced a period of chronic stress prior to the onset of cancer (Simonton and Mathews-

Simonton, 1980). In other words, he suggested that stress caused immunosuppression, thereby allowing cancer to flourish.

It appears that the level of immunosuppression is proportional to both the duration of stress and the level of stress. In contrast, deep relaxation has a positive effect on immune function. One particular research study showed that powerful immunity-enhancing chemicals are released in the body during periods of deep sleep (Moldofsky *et al.*, 1986). This supports what our common sense tells us – that deep relaxation and good-quality sleep counteract the effects of stress.

It is reasonable, therefore, to suggest that chronic stress, through its negative effects on immunity, can result in an increased susceptibility to cancer. Why, then, do some people exposed to ongoing stress get sick and others do not? In a study done at Carnegie Mellon University in the USA, 47 per cent of individuals under high levels of stress became ill, but what about the remaining 53 per cent (Cohen *et al.*, 1991)? The subject of how your mental state can affect your physical health is very interesting.

In 1989, Dr David Sobel and Dr Robert Orstein wrote a book entitled *Healthy Pleasures* in which they outlined details of their research on two groups of people, optimists and pessimists. They showed scientifically that optimists enjoy better immune function compared to pessimists. Optimists were shown to have higher numbers of one type of lymphocyte cell, which stimulates immune function. These cells are called helper cells. Pessimists, on the other hand, had higher numbers of cells that reduce immune function, called suppressor cells. The higher one's level of helper cells, the better one's resistance to disease; and the higher one's level of suppressor cells, the weaker one's resistance (Sobel and Ornstein, 1989).

Therefore, your state of mind can have a profound effect on your health. We know this intrinsically, but it is also nice to have it confirmed by science. It reinforces the fact that there is a very strong mind–body link. This is further illustrated by a study done on laboratory animals as regards the effects of hopelessness on health. From such studies it would appear that hopelessness not only predisposes you to the development of cancer but leads to more aggressive tumours (Visintainer *et al.*, 1982).

In this study, laboratory rats were divided into three groups and all three groups were injected with cancer cells. In group one, the rats received no electric shock. In group two, the rats were subjected to electric shocks but if they pressed a lever the shocks stopped. In group three, the rats received electric shocks but could do nothing to control these shocks. The group that did best was group two; because they had control of the situation, they fared better. The rats in group three fared worst of all because they had no control over their stressful environment.

This would suggest that the mind plays a major role in the outcome of the disease; a negative mindset *see*ms to promote it. This is why giving hope to people with cancer is so important. Dr Bernie Siegel, who I mentioned at the beginning of this chapter, advocates giving cancer patients hope. He has been accused of giving false hope, but his reply is that there is no such thing as false hope. I would agree with him.

Deep relaxation and meditation *see*m to have the opposite

effect of despair and hopelessness on the body. *You Can Conquer Cancer* is a great book written by a veterinary surgeon from Australia by the name of Ian Gawler. In it he describes how he developed bone cancer in his leg and had to have an amputation plus chemotherapy. Despite this aggressive treatment, the cancer spread throughout his body and his doctor gave him weeks to live. He decided to alter his diet radically and practise meditation for one hour three times a day. His cancer went into remission and he is still alive today (Gawler, 2001).

There are many stories along the same lines from all over the world. Most of them are centred on adopting a positive mindset combined with deep meditation. The power of meditation is enormous. It is one of the most effective anti-stress measures there is. When you are deeply relaxed, the whole functioning of your body alters.

STRESS AND DEEP-SEATED EMOTIONS

Research into ways in which your emotional state can affect your response to stress ranks **anger** as the single most powerful suppressor of immune function, predisposing you to a whole host of ailments. Dr Mara Julius of the University of Michigan looked at the effects of deep-seated anger on the health of women over an eighteen-year period. Each woman was asked to complete a questionnaire designed specifically to detect suppressed anger. The most startling aspect of this study was that women with a high score on the questionnaire – those with high levels of suppressed anger – were three times more likely to have died during the study period (eighteen years) compared to those with low levels of suppressed anger (Angier, 1990).

Many studies have since shown that anger can contribute to early death, heart disease and cancer.

In his book *Beyond Antibiotics*, Dr Michael A. Schmidt states that anger and hostility eat away at the substance of the human psyche. These emotions foster an atmosphere of negativity that clouds every human endeavour. I have heard some terrible stories over the past thirty years of physical, verbal or sexual abuse that engendered great anger in the victims.

I remember one patient in particular who came to *see* me with rather bizarre symptoms. When I enquired about her childhood, she said she could remember nothing. She had no memory before the age of sixteen. When I asked her for one happy memory from her childhood or a sad one, her memory bank was empty. This alarmed me and quickly it became apparent that her bizarre symptoms and lack of recollection of her childhood were a manifestation of some deep, deep trauma. I referred her to a psychiatrist who deals with childhood trauma by using visualisation and breathing techniques. Quickly we became aware that she had suffered severe abuse as a child. The abuse she had suffered had been so great that her only means of coping was to pretend it wasn't happening – hence the lack of memory.

I believe that the biggest advancement that can be made, not just for one's immunity but for one's whole body, is the release of anger. It not only benefits the individual but their family and loved ones as well as the wider community. I grew up in Northern Ireland and saw the effects of anger being released in a destructive way. I also attended a religious school and saw severe beatings being administered by teachers, which left us all traumatised.

I could list many case histories that I have recorded over the years but they all tell the same tale. Suppressed anger is one of the most destructive forces at work within the human being. Never underestimate the role of your emotions in controlling the state of your physical health. If you feel you have anger issues, do everything possible to release the anger in a constructive way, such as beating a punch bag or screaming into a pillow. Better still, consult a good psychologist or counsellor. You would be doing your immunity and your physical and emotional health in general a huge favour.

The positive release of anger not only benefits the individual but also their family and loved ones as well as the wider community.

THE ROLE OF FEAR

The biggest block to achieving your full potential in every walk of life is **fear.** So it follows that fear can be the biggest block to healing. Fear is part of the human condition and the game of life is about overcoming it. Fear has the power to cripple you and reduce you to total inactivity, or you can face your deepest fears and fight to overcome them. Often, facing your fears can have a powerful liberating experience and can allow you to follow your true path in life.

But before we can find our true destiny, it is necessary for us to be challenged by having to face our greatest fear; this is often referred to as 'the dark night of the soul'. Many years ago I was told by a very wise man that one's worst nightmare is one's greatest dream trying to come true. It has taken me many years and a very traumatic event to understand fully the truth of this saying.

Case History – Janet: Irritable Bowel Syndrome

Janet worked as a nurse in the Middle East and had been sent home because of ongoing bowel problems. Initially she was diagnosed as having parasites but despite treatment she did not improve. Her doctor then diagnosed her as having irritable bowel syndrome and said there was nothing further he could do. She then sought help from natural medicine and came to see me.

What became clear from talking to her was her skilful avoidance of answering questions relating to her feelings. She did not wish to talk about her emotional state, so I respected her wishes and began physical treatment to assist her bowel. I saw her frequently initially so that she got used to me; I hoped that at some point she would feel it safe to confide in me.

Two months later, after she had interrogated me sufficiently, she decided to open up and told me that she had been raped repeatedly by her uncle when she was quite young. Her uncle had died recently and she was now having nightmares about him. She had felt his presence in her bedroom on a few occasions.

This explained a lot about Janet – her need to check me out before confiding in me, her need to control everything in her life, her failure to have a normal relationship with a man. I used hypnosis to access the deep-seated fear that she lived with. It was only by bringing this fear from the subconscious mind to a conscious level that she began to see how it was pervading all aspects of her life.

I then referred her to a psychiatrist who used visualisation and breathing techniques to continue the healing. After months of treatment she had made significant progress to the point where she wanted to train as a counsellor for the Rape Crisis Centre. I find it interesting that those who have

experienced great difficulties, especially of an emotional
nature, end up being of great help in healing others who have
suffered similar pain.

Fear is a powerful and pervasive force, but bringing it to a
conscious level and talking to someone you trust can be
extremely therapeutic. This has been borne out by research
conducted at Stanford Medical School in California. This
study looked at a group of people who had cancer with
secondary tumours and who had a limited period of time
to live; these people were being forced to face their fear and
were therefore precisely the group of people needed for the
study.

The researchers wanted to assess the psychological
benefit of sharing experiences and feelings by getting the
group to meet once a week. The control group used for the
study was composed of people who also had cancer with
secondary tumours, but this group did not meet once a
week. The objective was to compare the two groups in the
hope that talking about fear of death would prove to be
therapeutic. Little did the researchers realise what a powerful effect it would have on the physical well-being of the
cancer patients involved.

The group that met once a week lived twice as long as the
control group. Those who attended the meetings regularly
lived longer than those who attended less frequently. In
fact, the more regularly a group member attended the
meetings, the longer he or she lived. These results were
published in *The Lancet* in 1989 and shocked the medical
world as they confirmed in clear terms the existence of a
mind–body connection (Spiegel *et al.*, 1989).

This study also confirmed that no matter how dire your prognosis, there is hope. By facing the fear of death, these patients showed it was possible to alter the outcome very significantly. Ten years after the study began, three of the patients in the group that met weekly were still alive, which is amazing considering they had advanced cancer and were given months to live at the time the study began. None of the patients in the control group was alive ten years later (Spiegel *et al.*, 2007).

Fear generates hormones that suppress your immune system. Simply talking about fear boosts the immune system. Clearly, this research paved the way for counselling to become an integral part of treatment, not just for cancer but for a whole host of conditions precipitated by stress. It also paved the way for research on the benefits of counselling for other conditions.

Because of this ground-breaking research, the mind–body connection has been put in the scientific spotlight. It went from hocus-pocus status to hard scientific data. No longer could we deny the very significant role that emotions play in our lives. Concepts such as releasing anger and confronting fear have been accepted by even the most sceptical of researchers, and patients have been given permission to transform themselves from fearful mice into mighty mice.

EMOTIONS AND IMMUNITY

There are two basic energies or emotions that affect all of us – love and fear. These two energies affect us at our core or soul level. They are also mutually exclusive in that you can't experience the two simultaneously. Minute by minute, hour by hour, day by day, these are the forces that drive us. Out of love for our family we go to work and earn money to provide shelter and food. But fear of starvation can also be a driving force behind earning money. Many of our actions are driven either by fear or by love.

Fear generates anxiety, and anxiety leads us to have negative thoughts and tense muscles, and to clench and grind our teeth. It also leads to the release of hormones that have a direct effect on the immune system. So, emotions have far-reaching effects in the body and often underlie immune-related illnesses such as cancer. Therefore, to prevent cancer it is necessary to confront any fear you may have by bringing it out of your subconscious into your conscious mind and then sharing it in a safe, protected space, with a close friend, partner, family member, therapist, etc. Once you deal with the fear it will have less power over your thoughts and actions, as in Janet's case above.

I refer my patients to a very wise man who has been trained as a psychiatrist but uses natural methods to help people. He does not use drug therapy but rather counselling, breathing techniques and visualisation. He has transformed the lives of a number of my patients. He is unique in the medical world. His name is Dr Pradeep Chadha and his website is: www.brclinicstresscentre.com.

At the National Cancer Institute in Washington, Dr Ronald Herberman and his associates showed that women who were better able to deal emotionally with the diagnosis of breast cancer had a much more active immune system – they had a higher number of killer T-cells, which attack and kill the cancer cells. (If you remember from Chapter 1, Mighty Mouse had a very active immune system in that he had a high number of killer cells, which were able to overcome the cancer cells.) Those who felt depressed and hopeless were shown to have much lower immune activity (Levy *et al.*, 1991).

This illustrates yet again the very strong connection between what you feel and your physical state of being. Your feelings affect your immunity and vice versa. The actual chemicals involved in this interaction have been identified – they are called neuropeptides. But how do you get from a negative place to a more positive one? How do you reduce the power of negative emotions and allow your immunity to protect you? Where do you start?

TALKING

If you are serious about preventing cancer developing in your body, talk to someone you trust about any emotional issues you may have and do so on a regular basis. Women are much better at this than men, but we men are beginning to learn. The power of just sitting in a room and talking is illustrated by this example from Northern Ireland. The famous psychologist Carl Jung visited Belfast, a very divided city, at the height of the Troubles in Northern Ireland. He chose four people each from the Catholic and Protestant communities who had lost loved ones because of the Troubles. He hired a hotel room for a weekend and allowed each person to express what they had experienced and how they felt. The sessions stopped only for eating and sleeping.

On Friday evening when the session began, there were obvious tensions between the two groups. By Sunday evening when the session ended, the eight people were close friends and hugged one another as they left. Through simply expressing their truths they were able to connect with each other and empathise with one another. Each of them went on to try to heal others in the community.

I remember *seeing* this as a documentary film in a lecture theatre in Trinity College in 1973. It had a profound effect on me as for the first time I saw a glimmer of hope for Northern Ireland. I also saw that, no matter how hopeless a situation appears to be, there is hope in simple solutions.

There is a very true expression in English: a problem shared is a problem halved. The more you talk about your innermost fears and feelings, the lighter you become and the healthier you become. Start by talking. When you have done that, move on to deep relaxation.

DEEP RELAXATION

It is when we are deeply relaxed that healing occurs. If you cut yourself accidentally, most of the healing will happen when you are deeply relaxed or asleep. Chronic anxiety, an overactive mind, lack of sleep, stress and anything else that impairs your ability to relax deeply will slow the healing process, not just at a physical level but at all levels.

You don't have to focus your conscious mind on the cut to enable it to heal; it heals automatically as if by magic. Therefore healing is a natural process. Blocking this healing energy within oneself by being stressed, for example, is an unnatural process. Allow the magic of self-healing to take place by creating a space and time for your body to relax deeply. First thing in the morning or last thing at night are perhaps the best times to do this. Personally, I prefer sunrise and sunset as these are the high energy points of the day.

There are many ways to relax deeply, from focusing on your breathing to focusing on releasing tension from different parts of the body through to self-hypnosis. The key with all of these techniques is to calm yourself physically and mentally so that you can open up at a deeper level.

BREATHING

It is possible to control stress building up in your body through controlling the way you breathe. Focusing your attention on your breathing to the exclusion of everything else can have a calming effect; it can be an extremely simple and effective tool to reduce stress levels. It is possible to do this anywhere at any time and has a proven benefit.

During periods of stress, the rate of breathing alters, as does the depth of breathing. Because of a high output of adrenalin at these times, your breathing becomes more rapid and much shallower, and you may have to take a deep breath occasionally to increase the oxygen level in your bloodstream. People who are chronically stressed can often cope much better if they are taught to take control of their breathing. Here is a simple exercise that works well.

Breathing Exercise

The purpose of this exercise is to breathe from your abdomen and to build up the level of carbon dioxide in your bloodstream, which has a relaxant effect.

Step 1: Push your tummy out as you begin inhaling, and when your tummy is fully expanded start using your chest to complete the in-breath.

Step 2: Practise this for a few minutes. When you can do it with ease, inhale slowly through your nose. Then hold your breath for five seconds and exhale quickly through the mouth, expelling as much air as possible. Do this three times.

Step 3: Take ten normal breaths, remembering to use your abdomen.

Step 4: Repeat step two, but hold your breath for seven seconds instead of five seconds.

Step 5: Breathe normally again.

The more you practise this exercise, the more effective it will be at calming you down. This is a very simple way of using your own power to reduce your levels of stress hormones, so protecting your immunity.

Breathing is another example of the mind–body link. Controlling your breathing has an immediate calming effect on your mind as well as on your body, so that your thoughts are not racing and are more focused. Breathing also connects body and soul. In many languages the word for breath also means spirit and this is where we get the word 'respiration' from.

Breathing connects the voluntary and involuntary parts of the nervous system (the adrenaline–noradrenaline system), as well as connecting the subconscious mind with the conscious mind. Breathing is therefore extraordinarily special. Buddhist monks learn the art of meditation by first focusing on their breathing since this can alter one's level of consciousness – slow, deep breathing allows one to access the deeper levels of one's being.

By getting into the routine of doing this you will then be able to progress to silent meditation, which is the most powerful healing tool available to all of us. It is the king of healing modalities, which is the reason why millions of people worldwide practise it on a regular basis. It is the best antidote to stress.

SILENT MEDITATION

Because our Western way of life is packed full of activity, we seldom make time to balance this activity with periods of inactivity and silence. This balance is essential for the proper functioning of the nervous system and hormonal system – these two systems are nowadays referred to as the neuroendocrine system.

Sleep is a period of relative physical inactivity, but one's mind is still active, as are one's emotions. Indeed, some people are also physically active when asleep through sleep talking, sleepwalking, clenching and grinding teeth, etc. Silent meditation is the most effective way of balancing the neuroendocrine system.

While I was visiting a medical clinic in the USA many years ago, the doctor in charge demonstrated the effect of silent meditation on blood flow to the right and left sides of the brain. The patient being tested was a male business executive who was highly stressed. The electrodes attached to his head measured the blood flow to both hemispheres of his brain. At the beginning of the test there was a high blood flow to his left brain and little blood flowing into the right side. After thirty minutes of silent meditation, there was equal blood flow to both sides of his brain – that is the natural state. Therefore meditation had a very demonstrable effect on the blood supply to the man's brain and as a consequence on his brain activity; it led to balance between the two hemispheres.

The stress of modern life leads to an imbalance in the activity of the two sides of the brain, which in turn causes further stress on the more subtle aspects of our being. As a consequence, the caring, compassionate, intuitive, creative and loving side of our nature gets little expression. Because of social conditioning, men tend to have more extreme imbalances than women. Silent meditation is essential for us all, but it is men who would appear to be in greater need.

Through silent meditation we are able to withdraw from our busy lives and begin to gain insights into ourselves and how we are living our lives. The greater your understanding of your true self, the more comfortable you will feel and the happier you will be to express the truth of how you feel. In this way, you will find yourself and gain a deep peace and contentment; you will 'come home', so to speak.

When you come home and discover who you really are, there will be no need for any more role playing, game playing, pretending or lies. You can bring yourself to the world without fear. Getting to know, becoming intimate with and learning to love yourself is the only means to happiness and the only means to permanently overcome anxiety, fear, guilt, jealousy and a lack of anything in your life, such as money.

The more finely tuned in to yourself you are, the more finely tuned you will be to everyone and everything around you. You will sense the inner conflicts within people more acutely; you will sense their anger, fear and frustration more easily. Conversely, you will also *see* the beauty and love in people more readily and will feel the urge to help them recognise it as well.

Silent meditation is the key that unlocks the door to your soul, the real you. It is the single most important form of healing for people, irrespective of religion, background, race or level of awareness. Increasing your level of self-awareness is the way out of your difficulties. If each of us practises the art of silent meditation regularly, there is definite hope for humanity. Try to practise meditation for at least thirty minutes daily and try to encourage the rest of your family to practise with you.

NUTRITION AND STRESS

Stress depletes the body of certain vitamins and minerals. Adrenalin speeds up your metabolism, resulting in a more rapid conversion of glucose into energy. To convert glucose to energy, B vitamins and magnesium are required. As a consequence, during periods of stress, high levels of B vitamins, magnesium, potassium and zinc are important, so if you feel under pressure in your life use a good vitamin and mineral supplement.

Replenish vitamins and minerals by eating lots of legumes, vegetables and fruit, and reduce sugary foods and refined carbohydrate, especially white flour. I discuss diet in detail in Chapters 5 and 6.

Some herbs such as ginseng and liquorice help to nourish and strengthen the adrenal glands and protect them during times of stress. These herbs are called adaptogens as they help you adapt to or cope with stress. They alter the hormonal response to stress and provide the body with more energy.

Ginseng

Ginseng protects the body from the harmful effects of stress; it also protects against physical and mental fatigue. It is the best herb to take to support adrenal gland function.

There are many studies that demonstrate ginseng's anti-stress activity. They show how ginseng can assist with extremely stressful conditions, improving mental alertness and athletic performance. It can be taken as a liquid extract or in dried form as a powder. I personally prefer to use it as a powder when I experience periods of stress. I combine it with liquorice to assist its absorption into the bloodstream. I use a quarter teaspoon of ginseng with the same amount of liquorice mixed together in a little water.

Liquorice

I am quite sure you are familiar with liquorice as it is used in the manufacture of certain sweets such as Liquorice Allsorts. The root of the liquorice plant has medicinal properties that have been recognised for centuries. It not only assists the adrenal glands but has many other interesting functions.

First, it is known to be antiviral and antibacterial and so is used to treat a range of infections. Liquorice is also added to a lot of cough mixtures. It is most commonly used by herbalists and other natural health practitioners to treat respiratory complaints. It can loosen congestion, making it much easier to clear phlegm; it's also used for sore throats and hoarseness.

What is of greater interest is the fact that the National Cancer Institute in Washington is investigating its use as an anti-cancer herb. It has definite anti-oestrogen activity, making it suitable for use as a protective agent against hormonal cancers. However, its anti-inflammatory effects are of greater interest, making it suitable as a general anti-cancer agent.

It is best to combine liquorice with other adaptogens such as ginseng if you wish to protect your adrenal glands from the effects of chronic stress. Use ginseng and liquorice in equal amounts. However, if using liquorice, an issue to be aware of is that it has the ability to raise blood pressure. If you have blood pressure problems and still wish to use liquorice, then use a form of liquorice that is free of the compound glycyrrhizic acid. Solgar, for example, have a version that has had this compound removed and it should be available in your local health shop.

I would like to finish this chapter with an interesting patient who came to *see* me many years ago with an uncommon symptom associated with stress.

Case History – John: Anal Pain

John worked abroad in the stock exchange and was back in Ireland for a short visit. He came to see me complaining of tightness and pain in his anal sphincter, which made it very difficult for him to have a bowel motion. This problem was getting progressively worse and he was very worried about it. John had noticed that the condition improved when he went on holiday. More recently, he had experienced short bouts of heart palpitations intermittently throughout the day.

He described his job as very stressful as he was doing several tasks all at the same time. He also had to travel a considerable distance to and from work and was therefore away from home for more than thirteen hours per day.

I treated John by giving him relaxation exercises to do every day. I prescribed ginseng and a high-dose B complex supplement and suggested improvements to his diet. I also asked him to take up yoga or meditation. On this treatment, he improved a lot physically to the point where he could pass a motion with ease again and the palpitations had ceased.

Even more important, he became aware of what his stressful lifestyle was doing to him and decided to change his job. He also became aware of how important it was to spend more time with his young family. Fortunately, John was willing to change everything in his life to ease his symptoms. Illness had made him desperate.

An amazing change took place in this man because he was ready and willing to heal. Stress can be positive in that it can spur you to make meaningful changes. Sometimes we have to take the wrong road before we find the right one.

SUMMARY

After nutrition, stress is the next major causative factor in the huge increase in a range of cancers. Poor diet weakens your body generally, while stress weakens the immune system in particular. In hospital, doctors use steroids such as cortisol to deliberately suppress the immune system in patients who have undergone organ transplantation, for example. The very same hormone, cortisol, is produced by the body in response to stress.

If stress lasts for a short time, there are no damaging consequences or side effects. However, if stress is sustained over a long period, such as years, immune suppression ensues. You no longer resemble Mighty Mouse but rather 'Mini' Mouse, since you are unable to attack and destroy cancer cells.

There are obvious external stressors such as the death of a loved one that can be hard to cope with and that make us sad, anxious, depressed and stressed. What are often hidden from view are the internal stressors such as anger and fear. Acknowledging and dealing with these external and internal stressors is the first and major step, not just in preventing cancer, but in fulfilling your true potential as a human being.

If you have grown up in Western society, chances are you need to address stress issues. We Westerners are very physically and mentally active, but do not balance this with periods of deep relaxation. Almost everyone in the West needs to balance their lives to some extent. Learn a method of deep relaxation and practise it regularly. If you have been under stress or are experiencing it at present, then take supplements that help you cope, such as ginseng, liquorice and a good vitamin and mineral supplement. Liquorice is especially good as it has anti-cancer effects.

Chapter 9
The Role of Obesity

You are more than likely aware that obesity increases your risk of developing certain forms of cancer. Before examining the link between obesity and cancer, it is helpful to explore the issue of obesity in some detail.

Obesity is on the increase in the parts of the world where people consume Western food. All of us are aware that, as a people, we are more overweight than we were thirty years ago. Yet exactly how common is obesity? How many adults walking on the street do you think are overweight? How many adults do you think are obese?

In Ireland, 66 per cent of Irish men over the age of twenty are considered overweight or obese, as are 50.9 per cent of Irish women over twenty (www.rte.ie/news/ireland/2014/0529/620368-irelands-obesity-levels-above-eu-average). The figures are approximately the same in the UK and are worse in the USA.

As we progress through this epidemic, two things are becoming apparent:

1. More and more people are being affected.
2. Those who are already overweight are finding that their weight is increasing faster with time.

In other words, more of us are getting fat and those who are already fat are getting fatter faster and faster. Clearly this is not a story of putting on a few extra pounds and having difficulty losing it. This is a much more serious situation. It is about the breakdown of normal weight control mechanisms in the body, as the following case history shows.

Case History – James: Body Mass Index (BMI) 32

James was a 27-year-old man who came to me asking for help with his sleep problems and his overactive gut. He had been diagnosed with type 2 diabetes and was on medication to control his blood sugar levels. He told me that he had an insatiable appetite and never felt full. He was eating mostly burgers, chips, bread and pizza. He also drank lots of soft drinks, fruit juice and water. He had recently been diagnosed with high blood pressure and was taking medication for that as well.

James visited his doctor, who advised him to exercise and referred him to a dietician. The dietician recommended that he eat more fruit, vegetables, lean protein and low-fat dairy such as low-fat cheese and skimmed milk. James found it easy to exercise by playing tennis because he had always loved the game, but he found it difficult to follow the dietary advice since the extra exercise only increased his hunger pangs. He described himself as being addicted to carbohydrates and having no taste for fruit, vegetables or any of 'those other foods'. He just craved more and more starchy foods and soft drinks. When he did not consume them, he immediately began to feel withdrawal symptoms: cravings, depression and irritability. Eventually he would give in and eat starch, but then this would quickly escalate to binge eating as his withdrawal symptoms decreased with consumption. He felt trapped in this cycle of addiction and his doctor and dietician were not able to help him to escape it. Every day was a huge battle for James as his weight kept increasing, despite trying to follow his doctor's advice.

Recently he had begun to have sleeping problems; his partner told him he was mouth breathing, snoring and had sleep apnoea (temporarily stopping breathing while asleep) on occasion. This was what brought him to see me. I explained to him that I had to treat the root cause of his obesity.

I told him that certain substances in his diet were causing him to put on weight, which blocked certain hormones from functioning and induced all of his other difficulties. When he finally grasped what was wrong with his body's biochemistry, James realised what he had to do to fix it. Through making changes to his diet and the addition of nutritional supplements, between the two of us we managed to not only get him off all medications but also to decrease his BMI (measure of body fat based on height and weight) and ultimately return him to a normal, healthy weight.

James's story is very typical. For a few people, the advice to eat less and exercise more can work in the short term. Usually, however, hunger takes over and the person has to abandon treatment and so a vicious cycle of dieting and bingeing commences.

We are over thirty years into the obesity epidemic and it is clear that conventional medical advice is not working. The overweight are becoming obese and the obese are becoming morbidly obese, and more and more of the human population are being affected.

When did this obesity epidemic begin? The figures in Tables 9.1 and 9.2 can answer this question.

Table 9.1: Percentage of Men in Each BMI Category (UK), 1966–1999

Men	1966	1972	1982	1989	1999
BMI <18.5	2.3	1.9	1.3	0.6	0.3
BMI 18.5–24.9	83.7	72.6	54.7	44	27.9
BMI 25–29.9	12.8	23.0	37.8	44.7	49.2
BMI >30	1.2	2.7	6.2	10.6	22.6

Source: https://apps.who.int/infobase/Indicators.aspx.

Table 9.2: Percentage of Women in Each BMI Category (UK), 1966–1999

Women	1966	1972	1982	1989	1999
BMI <18.5	7.8	5.4	3.7	1.6	0.3
BMI 18.5–24.9	81.1	78.0	70.4	58.5	37.6
BMI 25–29.9	9.2	13.9	19.0	25.8	36.3
BMI >30	1.8	2.7	6.9	14.0	25.8

Source: https://apps.who.int/infobase/Indicators.aspx.

These figures apply to the UK. As you can *see* from Table 9.1, the percentage of men with normal weight – a BMI of 18.5 to 24.9 – dropped from almost 84 per cent to almost 28 per cent between 1966 and 1999. Also, the number of obese men – those who have a BMI above 30 – rose from 1.2 per cent in 1966 to 22.6 per cent in 1999. The same trend can be *see*n in the figures in Table 9.2, which relate to women in the UK.

However, what these figures also reveal, particularly Table 9.1, is that a very significant increase in the number of overweight (BMI 25–30) and obese people (a BMI of 30+ is considered obese) occurred after 1972. Something happened in the early 1970s to cause this significant increase.

As mentioned earlier in this book, in the early 1970s we were told that animal fat caused heart disease and so food manufacturers reduced the fat content of many products. Doing this rendered the food very bland and tasteless, so they replaced the fat with sugar. Low-fat foods are essentially high-sugar foods. No surprise, then, that the wide availability of processed food and drinks laden with sugar led to weight gain on a national and international scale.

Small amounts of sugar are relatively harmless, such as the amounts that I grew up with. Large amounts of sugar generate the production of fat in the liver. You can therefore end up with a fatty liver. Much of this fat enters the bloodstream and leads to the deposition of fat in many organs. This has serious consequences. It is why many obese people end up with clogged arteries, heart disease, diabetes and a range of other illnesses.

However, the biggest and most significant risk that we all face from the obesity epidemic is cancer. Let me explain why.

Obesity causes the deposition of fat in the liver which in turn can lead to liver cirrhosis. As we know from chronic alcoholism, cirrhosis can result in primary liver cancer. So, as more and more of us become overweight and obese, the incidence of primary liver cancer increases.

You can now *see* that losing weight is a very serious issue. It's not just about losing a few pounds but rather an issue of avoiding serious liver damage and liver cancer. But the risks associated with weight gain do not end there.

It is known that fat deposits generate the production of oestrogen, which is the reason why some overweight men develop breast tissue and end up with 'man boobs'.

As you now know, oestrogen is associated with various cancers, especially breast cancer and cancer of the womb (endometrial cancer).

In this context, you can *see* why there has been a huge increase in the incidence of certain cancers, such as breast cancer, since the mid-1970s. It has to with the fact that many more people have gained fat stores, which leads to the excess production of oestrogen. Too much oestrogen acts as a carcinogen on tissues that have oestrogen receptors, such as those of the womb and breast.

There is a clear link between obesity and liver cancer and between obesity and breast cancer and endometrial cancer. Therefore, as obesity increases, we should *see* more and more cases of these forms of cancer. As Figure 1.1 in Chapter 1 illustrates very well, the incidence of breast cancer has kept pace with the rise in obesity.

It is therefore imperative to keep your weight under control. I have outlined treatment for losing weight and discussed supplements that work and those that don't in my e-book *The Big Fat Secret*.

SUMMARY

Obesity is now being described in many textbooks as a pandemic as it is affecting most of the world. It began in the mid-1970s and has continued unabated since. If this trend continues, half of the population will be obese by 2050 and the other half will be overweight. The basic reason for this pandemic is the addition of huge amounts of sugar to many processed foods.

Obesity has been partly responsible for the increase in certain cancers, such as breast cancer, endometrial cancer, prostate cancer and primary liver cancer. Therefore, losing weight has important anti-cancer effects. According to the experts, all of us are slowly gaining weight, so we should act by reducing the amount of sugary foods and drinks in our diet.

Chapter 10
Practical Advice for Specific Cancers

In this chapter I am going to leave all the theory aside and focus on simple, practical measures you can take to avoid getting some of the more common cancers. Some of this advice you may be aware of already through various public health campaigns.

What I would like you to keep in mind, and what I've tried to show throughout this book, is that it is not only exposure to known carcinogens that will determine who develops cancer, but rather the state of your immune system. For example, I had a lot of exposure to patients with tuberculosis during the years I spent in Africa and patients with open or highly infective tuberculosis have coughed on me, yet I did not contract this infection. My immune system was obviously robust enough to cope with this repeated exposure.

However, having said that, you don't want to put your body in harm's way, such as by living close to a source of ionising radiation. We have to be practical and minimise exposure to anything that can weaken the body and impair our immunity. So, although exposure is not the main determinant in the development of cancer, you should reduce your exposure to known carcinogens where possible.

I shall now look at some of the more common cancers in the West and what you can do to reduce your risk of getting these cancers.

BREAST CANCER

There has been a huge increase in the incidence of breast cancer since the 1940s. Clearly this has nothing to do with genetics but rather with environmental changes. The two main factors involved in bringing about this huge increase are diet and hormone disrupters in the environment.

Therefore, if you wish to reduce your risk of breast cancer, make serious changes to your diet, including avoiding sugar, dairy produce and wheat flour, and introduce lots of phytoestrogens such as soya – *see* Chapter 5 for more specific details.

In addition to modifying your diet, check that your gut is digesting and absorbing food correctly. Also, become very familiar with chemicals in your environment that can disturb the hormonal system and avoid these where possible – *see* Chapter 2 for more details.

COLON CANCER

There are a number of major considerations when trying to prevent bowel (colon) cancer. First, it is extremely important to have a gut function test performed, as I discussed in Chapter 4. For example, if you eat animal protein and are unable to digest it correctly for whatever reason, then the protein will go off or decay in your bowel, producing very toxic chemicals and damaging the wall of the colon. Hence, it is really essential to test your digestive ability.

Another critical factor to consider is the health of the

bacterial population that lines the colon. A healthy bacterial population produces certain chemicals, called organic acids, which nourish the cells lining the colon and protect them. The most important organic acid produced by the bacterial flora is butyric acid. This organic acid forms the main food for the cells that line the bowel. Without sufficient butyric acid, these cells become inflamed and colitis begins. As you learned earlier in this book, chronic inflammation predisposes you to the development of cancer. Therefore, protecting the gut flora is very important if you wish to prevent colon cancer. Take a good bacterial supplement daily, such as the 'for daily wellbeing' formula by OptiBac Probiotics.

It is also a good idea to have a colonoscopy performed every few years if you are over the age of fifty and especially if there is a family history of bowel cancer. It's even more important to have this procedure done if there is a family history of polyps in the colon or you have had polyps removed from your colon previously. There is an increased incidence of cancer in those with either colitis or with polyps. Therefore, take both conditions seriously.

As regards diet, don't heed the arguments against eating animal protein. As I looked at in Chapters 3 and 5, the evidence suggests that casein, the main protein in milk, is indeed a promoter of cancer. However, I have argued that including milk in your diet is fine, as long as you take it in its raw, unpasteurised form. Organic animal protein should form part of your diet; it forms a large part of the diet of the Maasai in East Africa, the Fulani in West Africa and the Inuit in Greenland, and bowel cancer is not present among these peoples.

Another issue to be aware of in preventing bowel cancer is to avoid constipation, especially if you consume animal produce. Allowing waste to build up in the rectum and lower colon will irritate and inflame the bowel wall. This will predispose it to the growth of cancer. Therefore, take ground flax*seed* or flax*seed* oil. Flax*seed* is both a bulking agent, which will alleviate constipation, and an anti-inflammatory, which will ease any inflammation in the colon.

LUNG CANCER

Lung cancer is by far the most common form of cancer in many countries, especially where a large section of the population smoke cigarettes. The huge increase in incidence in many Western countries during the twentieth century is directly related to cigarette smoking. Initially, lung cancer was more common in men, but as women took up the smoking habit, they too began to suffer. It now ranks as the most common cancer in men and women and has been so for almost fifty years; it is also the most common cause of cancer deaths.

It is obvious that the single most important way to prevent lung cancer is to not smoke and to avoid other people's cigarette smoke. Fortunately, in many Western countries smoking in public places has been banned.

It is interesting to note that, while smoking is very common in many Asian countries, the incidence of lung cancer is much lower than in the West. It is now thought that certain elements of the Asian diet are playing a protective role. Most attention has been focused on green tea, which is consumed in large quantities in countries such as China, and which is known to block the spread of cancer by blocking the formation of new blood vessels (*see* Chapter 5). Therefore, in addition to giving up smoking, try drinking green tea every day as a way of preventing, not just lung cancer, but many other cancers as well.

Another good preventive measure is to have your home and workspace checked for radon gas, as this is strongly associated with lung cancer. As you learned in Chapter 2, radon gas is formed by the radioactive decay of uranium in the soil. Because it is invisible and odourless, it is very hard to detect. A special metre has to be installed in your home to detect the presence of this gas. Contact the Environment Protection Agency and they will supply you with a kit plus further information. In the interim, make sure your house is very well ventilated.

Other possible causes of lung cancer include breathing in noxious fumes from car exhausts or industrial processes. There are laws in many countries to prevent occupational exposure to toxic fumes and, as a result, this cause of lung cancer is now rare. It is wise to wear an industrial mask if there is any possibility of exposure.

PROSTATE CANCER

As with breast cancer in women, prostate cancer is not common among Asians who eat a traditional diet rich in soya, vegetables and green tea and devoid of dairy products. Once Asian men adopt a Western diet, their chances of getting prostate cancer increase markedly.

Like breast cancer, prostate cancer is hormone related, so plant oestrogen will exert a protective effect, such as that in tofu, miso (seasoning made from soya beans), soya milk, soya yoghurt and soya plant. Diet plays a very important role in both protection against and the treatment of prostate cancer. Avoid dairy products and all refined food, such as cakes, biscuits, doughnuts and wheat breads, and avoid all sugary food and drinks.

Learn about hormone disrupters in the environment, such as plastics, pesticides and body-care products, and avoid these as much as possible (*see* Chapter 2). In that way you will minimise your risk of getting prostate cancer.

LEUKAEMIA, LYMPHOMA AND MULTIPLE MYELOMA (BLOOD CANCERS)

These cancers are grouped together as blood cancers. They affect the bone marrow or the lymph glands of the body. For the most part we do not know their causes but there are some clear associations.

First, there is a definite link between exposure to ionising radiation (*see* Chapter 2) and leukaemia. This became apparent after the atomic bomb was dropped on two Japanese cities, Hiroshima and Nagasaki, towards the end of the Second World War. Many of the survivors went on to develop leukaemia. This was not the first time a link had been made between leukaemia and ionising radiation. The main form of treatment for ankylosing spondylitis (an inflammatory disease that can cause the vertebrae in your spine to fuse together) was radiotherapy, and there was an increase in the incidence of leukaemia in patients treated in this way.

Therefore, to protect yourself from leukaemia, be careful about exposing yourself to too many X-rays and avoid CAT scans, except as a last resort. Learn about the various forms of ionising radiation, especially radon gas, and avoid where possible (*see* Chapter 2).

Second, there is also a link between exposure to toxic chemicals and metals and blood cancers. For example, it is known that exposure to benzene or petrol products may lead to leukaemia. Exposure to very toxic metals such as mercury and lead has been implicated in some blood cancers as well. The International Agency for Research on Cancer has classified lead as a probable carcinogen, based on animal and human studies.

Your water supply still remains your main source of exposure to lead. Therefore, use bottled water or get a filter that will remove metals from the water supply. Distillation units are particularly good as they remove everything from the water, including chemicals and metals.

Third, blood cancers can be associated with certain viruses, similar to the viruses that cause leukaemia in cats and cattle. Therefore, like Mighty Mouse, you can boost your immunity and prevent viruses from multiplying in the cells of your body. Once again, diet is important here (*see* Chapter 5), as are anti-stress measures (*see* Chapter 8).

Fourth, there is growing evidence that aspartame, the artificial sweetener, may be responsible for blood cancer. It is sold under the trade names Equal and NutraSweet.

It is also used to sweeten a whole host of products from soft drinks to medicines. A study by a doctor working in one of the teaching hospitals associated with Harvard Medical School, and published in the *American Journal of Clinical Nutrition* in December 2012, showed a link between aspartame consumption in humans and blood cancers such as lymphoma, multiple myeloma and leukaemia

(Schernhammer *et al.*, 2012). Previous studies carried out by Italian researchers on laboratory animals also confirmed this cancer-forming ability of aspartame (Soffritti *et al.*, 2007).

To prevent exposure to aspartame, you will have to read the labels on food and medicine products as it is a very commonly used sweetener. Here is a brief list of some of the medicines and health products that contain it.

- Vitamin tablets, including those meant for children such as brands like Flintstones and Bugs Bunny
- Laxatives and bulking agents such as Maalox, Metamucil and Fybogel
- Antibiotics such as Augmentin and Amoxil
- Stomach medicines such as Zantac, Pepcid and Zoton
- Chest medicines such as Benadryl and Singulair
- Others such as Lemsip, Calcichew and Calpol

It is particularly worrying that some of these medicines are meant for children, such as Calpol, Benadryl and some vitamin tablets. My honest advice is to avoid all products that contain any artificial sweetener. Use products that contain natural sweeteners such as stevia or xylitol.

CERVICAL CANCER

This cancer is most commonly associated with infection of the cervix by the human papilloma virus. This virus can set up a chronic infection that can progress to cancer. It affects mostly middle-aged women but can occur in younger women. It is also more common in women who have had multiple childbirths. The reason for this may be that the trauma associated with childbirth can damage the cervix and set up a chronic inflammatory condition, which, as you know, is a risk factor for developing cancer.

Cervical cancer is also more common in women who have had many sex partners. The reason for this is that the human papilloma virus is sexually transmitted. Therefore, the greater the number of sexual partners you have, the higher your risk of being infected with the virus that causes cervical cancer.

The Pap smear, also called the Papanicolaou screening test or smear test, is the best way to check for cervical cancer. This simple test will usually detect the presence of any abnormal cervical cells. It is a very important preventive test for all women, but especially those who are sexually active and those who have had traumatic deliveries. Have a Pap smear done once a year so that any area of the cervix that may have abnormal cells can be treated promptly.

Another way of protecting yourself against the development of cervical cancer is to follow an anti-inflammatory diet (*see* Chapter 5).

TESTICULAR CANCER

Testicular cancer is not common, but when it does occur it is usually in men aged between eighteen and forty. It has featured in the news somewhat over the past few years, as some high-profile sportsmen, such as cyclist Lance Armstrong, have been diagnosed with it.

The testes produce the male hormone testosterone and so testicular cancer is hormone based. Anything that disrupts the production of testosterone in the body has the potential to cause testicular cancer.

One of the most common causes is an undescended testicle, which has a high risk of becoming malignant. This why doctors always check newborn male children to make sure that both testes have descended into the scrotum. If one or both have failed to descend it is possible to intervene surgically. This is important preventive medicine.

There are other causes, however, one of which relates to the use of hormones by professional athletes. Some professional athletes use hormones, especially testosterone, to increase body strength. When taken consistently over a number of years, these have the potential to cause disruption of the natural production of testosterone and so lead to cancer.

Other hormone disrupters such as pesticides and plastics (*see* Chapter 2) can also increase the risk of hormone-based cancers like testicular cancer.

To prevent testicular cancer, it is important to check that all male children have both testes in the scrotum. If you are a sportsman, do not use steroid supplements and avoid testosterone in particular. Also, avoid hormone disrupters in your environment as best you can.

LIVER CANCER

There are two types of liver cancer: primary liver cancer and secondary liver cancer.

Let's look at primary liver cancer first.

Primary Liver Cancer

This is cancer that develops in the cells of the liver itself. In other words, it has not spread from another site in the body. It occurs among populations in which there is a high carrier rate of the hepatitis virus – hepatitis B and C. Therefore, it is very uncommon in Western countries and really only found in parts of Africa and Asia. The virus is transmitted by sexual contact, via food and via other close contact with a carrier. The best protection is to use condoms and to be strict about good hygiene in the preparation of food.

Cirrhosis of the liver has more recently been recognised as a risk factor for the development of primary liver cancer. Cirrhosis of the liver is mainly associated with chronic alcoholics and the obese. Prevention obviously involves treatment for both of these conditions.

Secondary Liver Cancer

This is cancer that began in some other part of the body and has spread to the liver. The original cancer is referred to as the primary and the cancer found in the liver is referred to as the secondary. Almost any primary cancer, especially in the advanced stages, has the potential to spread to the liver via the bloodstream. The cancers that commonly lead to secondaries in the liver are bowel cancer, pancreatic cancer and stomach cancer, as well as advanced breast cancer. Prevention of secondary liver cancer has to do with treatment/prevention of the primary cancer.

SKIN CANCER (MELANOMA)

Melanoma is the malignant form of skin cancer and often begins in a pigmented mole or naevus. The people most at risk are the fair-skinned races, especially those who emigrate to sunnier countries, such as the Irish to Australia. The key to prevention is to protect the skin from excessive ultraviolet rays, either from the sun or from solariums (sunbeds).

If living in a sunny climate, wear protective clothing such as long trousers, long-sleeved shirts and broad-brimmed hats. If you can't avoid exposure to the sun, use sun cream with a high factor such as 30 plus. You often *see* cricketers using zinc ointment on their nose and lips as additional protection. This is only necessary where you will have prolonged exposure to the sun.

The other main preventative measure is to *see* a dermatologist as soon as you notice a change in a mole or naevus. Changes to be concerned about are: a change in size, a change in shape, a change in colour or a change to the surface of the mole, such as bleeding, scaliness, ulceration or itching. It is wise to report any change as soon as possible. The quicker you act, the better your chance of avoiding the spread of this cancer into the surrounding skin and systemically via the bloodstream.

CANCERS ASSOCIATED WITH SMOKING

Finally, I want to mention some of the cancers associated with cigarette smoking.

Most people are aware of the fact that lung cancer is caused by smoking cigarettes, but many are not aware of the many other cancers associated with this very addictive habit.

Cigarette smoke can cause a whole range of cancers, including mouth cancer, cancer of the lips, throat cancer, pancreatic cancer, stomach cancer, kidney cancer and bladder cancer. Quite a list! Smoking, or being a passive smoker, is very dangerous, which is the reason why so many countries have banned smoking in public spaces and have many public health warnings to inform people of the dangers.

If you wish to prevent cancer, do not smoke cigarettes, cigars, pipes, etc. Do not work or live where there is a risk of you being exposed to someone else's smoke. Also, warn your children about the dangers of smoking.

Bibliography

Aggarwal, B., Shishodia, S., Takada, Y., Banerjee, S., Newman, R.A., Bueso-Ramos, C.E. and Price, J.E, 'Curcumin suppresses the paclitaxel-induced nuclear factor pathway in breast cancer cells and inhibits lung metastasis of human breast cancer in nude mice', *Clinical Cancer Research*, 11(20), 2005: 7490–98.

Allen, N.E., Appleby, P.N., Davey, G.K., Kaaks, R., Rinaldi, S. and Key, T.J., 'The associations of diet with serum insulin-like growth factor 1 and its main binding proteins in 292 women meat-eaters, vegetarians and vegans', *Cancer Epidemiology, Biomarkers and Prevention*, 11(11), 2002: 1441–8.

Allen, N.E., Appleby, P.N., Davey, G.K., and Key, T.J., 'Hormones and diet: low insulin-like growth factor 1 but normal bioavailable androgens in vegan men', *British Journal of Cancer*, 83(1), 2000: 95–7.

Angier, N., 'Chronic anger is a major health risk: studies find', *New York Times*, 13 December 1990 (from papers presented at the 1990 conference of the American Heart Association).

Askling J., Linet, M., Gridley, G., Halstensen, T.S., Ekström, K. and Ekbom, A., 'Cancer incidence in a population-based cohort of individuals hospitalized with celiac disease or dermatitis herpetiformis', *Gastroenterology*, 123(5), 2002: 1428–35.

Azzouz, A., Jurado-Sánchez, B., Souhail, B. and Ballesteros, E., 'Simultaneous determination of 20 pharmacologically active substances in cow's milk, goat's milk and human breast milk by gas chromatography-mass spectrometry', *Journal of Agricultural and Food Chemistry*, 59, 2011: 5125–32.

Béliveau, R. and Gingas, D., *Foods that Fight Cancer*, New York: McClelland & Stewart, 2006.

Boik, J., *Natural Compounds in Cancer Therapy*, Princeton, MN: Oregon Medical Press, 2001.

Bryson, C., *The Fluoride Deception*, New York: Seven Stories, 2006.

Campaign for Safe Cosmetics and Environmental Working Group, 'Not So Sexy: The Health Risks of Secret Chemicals in Fragrance,' May 2010.

Campbell, C. and Campbell, T., *The China Study: The most comprehensive study of nutrition ever conducted and the startling implications for diet, weight loss and long term health*, Dallas: Benbella Books Inc., 2006.

Campbell, E.G., Weissman, J.S. and Ehringhaus, S. *et al.*, 'Institutional Academic-Industry Relationships', *Journal of American Medical Association*, 298(15), 2007: 1779–86.

Cao, Y. and Cao, R., 'Angiogenesis inhibited by drinking tea', *Nature*, 398(6726), 1999: 381.

Cohen, S., Tyrrell, D.A.J. and Smith, A.P., 'Psychological stress and susceptibility to the common cold', *New England Journal of Medicine*, 325, 1991: 606–12.

Cheng, A.L. *et al.*, 'Phase 1 clinical trial of curcumin, a chemopreventive agent, in patients with high-risk or pre-malignant lesions', *Anticancer Research*, 21(4B), 2001: 2895–900.

Cui, Z. *et al.*, 'Spontaneous regression of advanced cancer: identification of a unique genetically determined trait in mice', *Proceedings of the National Academy of Sciences* (USA), 100, 2003: 6682–7.

De Luca, L.M., 'Retinoids in differentiation and neoplasia', *Scientific American Science and Medicine*, July–August 1995: 28–36.

Demeule, M., Annabi, B., Michaud-Levesque, J., Lamy, S. and Bélieveau, R., 'Dietary prevention of cancer: anticancer and antiangiogenic properties of green tea polyphenols', *Medicinal Chemistry Reviews*, 2, 2005: 49–58.

Djamgoz, M. and Plant, J., *Beat Cancer*, London: Vermillion, 2014.

Dunn, S.E., Hardman, R.A., Kari, F.W. and Barrett, J.C., 'Insulin-like growth factor 1 (IGF-1) alters drug sensitivity of HBL100 human breast cancer cells by inhibition of apoptosis induced by diverse anti-cancer drugs', *Cancer Research*, 57(13), 1997: 2687–93.

Epstein, S., *The Politics of Cancer Revisited*, Fremont, NY: East Ridge Press, 1998.

Erasmus, U., *Fats that Heal, Fats that Kill*, Canada: Alive Books, 1993.

Falsaperla, M., Morgia, G., Tartarone, A., Ardito, R. and Romano, G., 'Support ellagic acid therapy in patients with hormone refractory prostate cancer (HRPC) on standard chemotherapy using vinorelbine and estramustine phosphate', *European eurology*, 474, 2005: 449–54.

Ferm, V.H., 'Arsenic as a teratogenic agent', *Environmental Health Perspectives*, 19, 1977: 215–17.

Gawler, I., *You Can Conquer Cancer – Prevention and Treatment*, South Yarra, Australia: Michelle Anderson Publishing, 2001.

Gray, A., Read, S., McGale, P. and Darby, S., 'Lung cancer deaths from indoor radon and the cost effectiveness and potential of policies to reduce them', *British Medical Journal*, 338, 2009: a3110.

Grothey, A., Voigt, W., Schöber, C., Müller, T., Dempke, W. and Schmoll, H.J., 'The role of insulin-like growth factor 1 and its receptor in cell growth, transformation, apoptosis, and chemoresistance in solid tumors', *Journal of Cancer Research and Clinical Oncology*, 125(3), 1999: 166–73.

Hara, M. *et al.*, 'Cruciferous vegetables, mushrooms and gastrointestinal cancer risks in a multicenter, hospital-based case-control study in Japan', *Nutrition and Cancer*, 46(2), 2003: 138–47.

Hardell, L. and Carlberg, M., 'Mobile phones, cordless phones and the risk for brain tumours', *International Journal of Oncology*, 35(1), 2009: 5–17.

Harris, R.E., Kasbari, S. and Farrar, W.B., 'Prospective study of nonsteroidal anti-inflammatory drugs and breast cancer', *Oncology Reports*, 6(1), 1999:71–73.

Harvey, G., *We Want Real Food: Why Our Food Is Deficient in Minerals and Nutrients – and What We Can Do About it*, London: Robinson, 2008.

Hibbeln, J., Lands, W. and Lamoreaux, E., 'Quantitative changes in the availability of fats in the us food supply', 5th Congress of the International Society for the Study of Fatty Acids and Lipids, Montreal, 7–11 May 2002: 10.

Ingram, D., 'Diet and subsequent survival in women with breast cancer', *British Journal of Cancer*, 69(3), 1994: 592–5.

International Agency for Research on Cancer, *Wood Dust and Formaldehyde*, IARC Monographs on the Evaluation of Carcinogenic Risks to Humans, 62, 1995.

Jankun, J. Selman, S.H., Swiercz, R. and Skrzypczak-Jankun, E., 'Why drinking green tea could prevent cancer', *Nature* 387(6633), 1997: 561.

Jenkins, D.J.H. Wolever, T.M., Taylor, R.H., Barker, H., Fielden, H., Baldwin, J.M., Bowling, A.C., Newman, H.C., Jenkins, A.L. and Goff, D.V., 'Glycaemic index of foods: a physiological basis for carbohydrate exchange', *American Journal of Clinical Nutrition*, 34(3), 1981: 362–6.

Karin, M. and Greten, F.R., 'NF-kB: linking inflammation and immunity to cancer development and progression', *Nature Reviews Immunology*, 5, 2005: 749–59.

Kidd P.M., 'The use of mushroom glucans and proteoglycans in cancer treatment', *Alternative Medical Review*, 5(1), 2000: 4–27.

King, M.C., Marks, J.H. and Mandell, J.B., 'Breast and ovarian cancer risks due to inherited mutations', *Science*, 302(5645), 2003: 643–6.

Levy, S.M., Herberman, R.B., Lippman, M., D'Angelo, T. and Lee, J., 'Immunological and psychosocial predictors of disease recurrence in patients with early-stage breast cancer', *Behavioural Medicine* 17(2), 1991: 67–75.

Lichtenstein, P., Holm, N.V., Verkasalo, P.K., Lliadou, A., Kaprio, J., Koskenvuo, M., Pukkala, E., Skytthe, A. and Hemminki, D., 'Environmental and heritable factors in the causation of cancer: analyses of cohorts of twins from Sweden, Denmark, and Finland', *New England Journal of Medicine*, 343(2), 2000: 78–85.

Long, L., Navab, R. and Brodt, P., 'Regulation of the $M\hat{r}$ 72,000 type IV collagenase by the type 1 insulin-like growth factor receptor', *Cancer Research*, 58(15), 1998: 3243–7.

McKenna, J.E., *Antibiotics: Are They Curing Us or Killing Us?* Dublin: Gill & Macmillan, 2014.

McKenna, J.E., *Good Food: Can You Trust What You Are Eating?* Dublin: Gill & Macmillan, 2013.

McKenna, J.E., *The Big Fat Secret: What they don't want us to know about why we're all gaining weight* (Kindle), 2012.

McKenna, J.E, *Natural Alternatives to Antibiotics*, Dublin: New Leaf Publishing Group, 2003.

McKenna, J.E., *Hard to Stomach: Real Solutions to Your Digestive Problems*, Dublin: New Leaf Publishing Group, 2002.

McLaughlin, N., Annabi, B., Lachambre, M.P., Kim, K.S., Bahary, J.P., Moumdjian, R. and Beliveau, R., 'Combined low dose ionising radiation and green tea-derived epigallocatechin-3-gallate treatment induces human brain endothelial cell death', *Journal of Neuro-Oncology*, 80(2), 2006: 111–21.

Marnewick, J.L., van der Westhuizen, F.H., Joubert, E., Swanevelder, S., Swart, P. and Gelderblom, W.C., 'Chemoprotective properties of rooibos (*Aspalathus linearis*), honeybush (*Cyclopia intermedia*) herbal and green and black (*Camellia sinensis*) teas against cancer promotion induced by fumonisin B1 in rat liver', *Food and Chemical Toxicology*, 47(1), 2009: 220–9.

Marnewick, J.L., Rautenbach, F., Venter, I., Neethling, H., Blackhurst, D.M., Wolmarans, P. and Macharia, M., 'Effects of rooibos (*Aspalathus linearis*) on oxidative stress and biochemical parameters in adults at risk for coronary artery disease', *Journal of Ethnopharmacology*, 133(1), 2011: 46–52.

Marx, J. 'Inflammation and cancer: the link grows stronger', *Science*, 306(5698), 2004: 966–8.

Mehta, K., Pantazis, P., McQueen, T. and Aggarwal, B.B., 'Antiproliferative effect of curcumin (*diferuloylmethane*) against human breast tumor cell lines', *Anticancer Drugs*, 8(5), 1997: 470–81.

Melia, P., 'One in ten homes at risk from lead in water', *Irish Independent*, 19 September 2014.

Moldofsky, H. , Lane, F.A., Eisen, J., Keystone, E. and Gorczynski, R.M., 'The relationship of Interleukin–1 and immune functions to sleep in humans', *Psychosomatic Medicine*, 48, 1986: 309–15.

Muncke, J., 'Endocrine disrupting chemicals and other substances of concern in food contact materials: an updated review of exposure, effect and risk assessment', *Journal of Steroid Biochemistry & Molecular Biology*, 127, 2011: 118–27.

National Council on Radiation Protection and Measurements, *Ionizing Radiation Exposure of the Population of the United States*, NCRP report no. 160, 3 March 2009.

National Research Council, *Diet and Health: Implications for Reducing Chronic Disease Risk*, Washington: National Academic Press, 1989: 376–9.

Nelson, J.E. and Harris, R.E., 'Inverse association of prostate cancer and non-steroidal anti-inflammatory drugs (NSAIDS): results of a case-control study', *Oncology Reports*, 7(1), 2000: 169–70.

Nordberg, G.F., *Handbook on the Toxicology of Metals*, London: Elsevier B.V., 2007.

O'Doherty, C., '30,000 homes at risk of lead poisoning from water', *Irish Examiner*, 3 January 2013.

Ontario College of Family Physicians, 'Review of research on the effects of pesticides on human health', 2012, www.ocfp.on.ca.

Ornish, D.M. *et al.*, 'Changes in prostate gene expression in men undergoing an intensive nutritional and lifestyle intervention', *Proceedings of the National Academy of Sciences*, 105(24), 2008: 8369–74.

Rubin, T. 'Make a splash with rooibos tea', *Better Nutrition*, February, 2010: 48–9.

Schernhammer, E., Bertrand, K.A., Birmann, B.M., Sampson, L., Willett, W.C. and Feskanich, D., 'Consumption of artificial sweetener- and sugar-containing soda and risk of lymphoma and leukemia in men and women', *American Journal of Clinical Nutrition*, 96, 2012: 1419–28.

Schmidt, M.A., *Beyond Antibiotics: Strategies for Living in a World of Emerging Infections and Antibiotic-Resistant Bacteria*, Berkeley, US: North Atlantic Books, 2009.

Selye, H., *Stress in Health and Disease*, London: Butterworths, 1976.

Servan-Schreiber, D., *Anti-Cancer: A New Way of Life*, London: Michael Joseph, 2011.

Shils, M.E., Olson, J.A. and Shike, M., *Modern Nutrition in Health and Disease*, Philadelphia: Lea & Febiger, 1994.

Siegel, B., *Love, Medicine and Miracles: Lessons Learned about Self-Healing from a Surgeon's Experience with Exceptional Patients*, New York: William Morrow Paperbacks, 1998.

Simonton, C. and Mathews-Simonton, S., *Getting Well Again*, London: Bantam, 1980.

Sobel D. and Ornstein, R., *Healthy Pleasures*, Massachusetts: Addison-Wesley, 1989.

Soffritti, M., Belpoggi, F., Tibaldi, E., Degli Esposti, D. and Lauriola, M., 'Lifespan exposure to low doses of aspartame beginning during prenatal life increases cancer effects in rats', *Environmental Health Perspectives*, 115, 2007: 1293–7.

Sommella, A., Deacon, C., Norton, G., Pigna, M., Violante, A. and Meharg, A.A., 'Total arsenic, inorganic arsenic, and other elements concentrations in Italian rice grain varies with origin and type', *Environmental Pollution*, 181, October, 2013: 38–43.

Spiegel, D. *et al.*, 'Effects of supportive–expressive group therapy on survival of patients with metastatic breast cancer', *Cancer*, 110(5) 2007: 1130–8.

Spiegel, D., Bloom, J.R., Kraemer, H.C. and Gottheil, E., 'Effect of psychosocial treatment on survival of patients with metastatic breast cancer', *Lancet*, 2(8673), 1989: 1209–10.

Stewart, B.W. and Kleihues, P. (eds), who *World Cancer Report*, Lyon: IARC Press, 2003.

Sugawara, G., Nagino, M. and Nishio, H., 'Perioperative symbiotic treatment to prevent postoperative infectious complications in biliary cancer surgery: a randomized controlled trial', *Annals of Surgery*, 244(5), 2006: 706–14.

Theunissen, I., 'Rooibos, the healthy tea', *Science in Africa*, March 2005.

Thun, M.J. 'nsaid use and decreased risk of gastrointestinal cancers', *Gastroenterology Clinics of North America*, 25(2), 1996: 333–48.

Tsubono, Y., Tsugane, S. and Gey, K.F., 'Plasma antioxidant vitamins and carotenoids in five Japanese populations with varied mortality from gastric cancer', *Nutrition and Cancer*, 34(1), 1999: 56–61.

Visintainer, M.E., Volpicelli, J.R. and Seligman, M.E.P., 'Tumor rejection in rats after inescapable or escapable shock', *Science*, 216, 1982: 437–9.

Wagner, M. and Oehlmann, J., 'Endocrine disrupters in bottled mineral water: estrogenic activity in the E-screen', *Journal of Steroid Biochemistry and Molecular Biology*, 127(1–2), 2011: 128–35.

Warburg, O., 'On the origin of cancer cells', *Science*, 123(3191), 1956: 309–14.

Waterhouse, J., Muir, C., Shanmugaratnam, K., and Powell, J., *Cancer Incidence in Five Continents, Vol. IV*, Lyon, France: WHO-IARC, 1982.

West, J., Logan, R.F.A., Smith, C.J., Hubbard, R.B. and Card, T.R., 'Malignancy and mortality in people with coeliac disease: a population-based cohort study', *British Medical Journal* 329, 21 July 2004: 716–19.

White, S.J., *The Extra Virgin Kitchen*, Dublin: Gill & Macmillan, 2014.

Yakymenko, I., and Sidorik, E., 'Risks of carcinogenesis from electromagnetic radiation of moblie telephony devices', *Experimental Oncology*, 329(2), 2010: 54–60.

Zhou, J., Yu, L., Mai, Z. and Blackburn, G.L., 'Combined inhibition of estrogen-dependent human breast carcinoma by soy and tea bioactive components in mice', *International Journal of Cancer*, 108(1), 2004: 8–14.

Index